Global Burnout

Thinking|Media

Series Editors:
Bernd Herzogenrath
Patricia Pisters

Global Burnout

Pascal Chabot
Translated from the French by Aliza Krefetz

Bloomsbury Academic
An imprint of Bloomsbury Publishing Inc

B L O O M S B U R Y
NEW YORK • LONDON • OXFORD • NEW DELHI • SYDNEY

Bloomsbury Academic
An imprint of Bloomsbury Publishing Inc

1385 Broadway
New York
NY 10018
USA

50 Bedford Square
London
WC1B 3DP
UK

www.bloomsbury.com

BLOOMSBURY and the Diana logo are trademarks of Bloomsbury Publishing Plc

This translated edition published by Bloomsbury Academic 2018
First published in French by Presses Universitaires de France 2013

Library of Congress Cataloging-in-Publication Data
A catalog record for this book is available from the Library of Congress

ISBN: HB: 978-1-501-33438-2
ePDF: 978-1-501-33440-5
eBook: 978-1-501-33439-9

Cover design: Daniel Benneworth-Gray
Cover image © Paolo Sanfilippo

Series: thinking|media

Typeset by RefineCatch Limited, Bungay, Suffolk
Printed and bound in the United States of America

To those who contemplate.

"If your only tool is a hammer, every problem looks like a nail"

Paul Watzlawick, *Change*

Contents

Foreword

The phenomenon we call burnout is not just a personal problem that affects a few exhausted individuals. It holds up a mirror to dysfunctions in the relationships between human beings and their material environment.

After analyzing the origins of the concept, the author identifies three main types of burnout: the first, specific to professions centered on caring for others, seems to stem from the exhaustion of their humanism; the second appears to be a problem of adaptation and perfectionism, while the third is a consequence of the struggle for recognition.

The philosophical implications of each of these three conditions are identified. Finally, burnout is presented as an occasion to rethink the pact between humanity and technology, and to reinterpret the notion of progress.

Introduction

Something is happening

Something is happening.

In the highway breakdown lane, a woman sits weeping in her car. It's strange, the way her tears seem to pour out uncontrollably. Nothing can stop them. It is as if her entire body were emptying itself, as if it were expelling a humor that cannot be contained. Her hands tremble. She rocks back and forth. And the look in her eyes is one of incomprehension mixed with fear.

Tears, they say, wash the emotions clean. But her tears aren't washing anything away. They are tears of destruction. A surge of suffering is ravaging an otherwise stable person. It is as if her very existence has overwhelmed her. This body, this car, this life, everything, suddenly seems to her useless and insurmountable.

We could understand this breakdown if it had happened in response to a death, a break-up, even a war. But there is no apparent cause for this implosion.

Something else is happening; for example, that haggard man in his forties. For the last hour, he has been sitting motionless in front of his computer. Mouth open, eyes wild, he seems to be frozen in place. Earlier, he was double-checking some numbers on a spreadsheet.

Then everything went black, leaving a gaping void, a vacantness that bordered on madness.

When he tried to get up, his body refused to obey him. From his pelvis to his shoulders, an inexplicable stiffness paralyzed his spine. He had to be taken away in an ambulance, in front of his stupefied co-workers. For three months now, he has been confined to his bed, suspended in a twilight zone between sleep and wakefulness. This man, who used to check his email every ten minutes, begins to tremble uncontrollably when his company's name is mentioned.

Strange things are happening, and it is the intention of this book to demonstrate that they constitute a philosophical concern, and that through the lens of philosophy we must try to understand them and situate them in our current age of excess.

Burnout is not just a problem experienced by isolated individuals. It seems, rather, to be connected to concepts of progress, technology, and desire, which are the hallmarks of this era of experimentation. There is a strange freneticism in the air, at once troubling and exciting. We are being modified by our own tools. The system leaves its mark on our thoughts and our expectations.

Burnout gives expression to the anxieties of our age. Astonishment is the fundamental basis of all philosophy. And nothing could be more astonishing than the contrast, in these two case studies, between the ordinary, seemingly pleasant lives of those afflicted and the intensity of their anguish. Because that woman weeping at the steering wheel and that executive paralyzed in front of his computer represent the most faithful followers of twenty-first century values. Educated university graduates, enthusiastic workers, they are the zealous supporters of our contemporary way of life. It is their tireless work—in excess of forty hours each week—that keeps the system in place. And yet they are the ones who crack.

Burnout is a disease of civilization. And civilization is bleeding the earth dry. We have transformed the biosphere into a resource. Our attitude toward nature is no longer contemplative but exploitative; we look for anything that could bring us profit, and in the process, we leave our imprint on the entire planet.

Nowadays, this exhaustion of resources is taking on a new dimension. It has begun to affect people, even those in the West who seemed to be safely removed from the negative impact of development. Those in charge are themselves falling victim to the mentality of exploitation. This comes as no surprise for some: the logic of techno-capitalism is global, and its consequences must therefore be universal. For others, however, it comes as a shock. Because they had been promised a better world. In the writing of certain ideologues of the 1960s, one is struck by the climate of optimism that surrounded technological development. Machines would liberate us from labor. They would toil in our stead. They would allow us to reclaim time, that supreme commodity. Ours would be a civilization built on leisure, a reconfiguration of the myth of an earthly Paradise, with automobiles and sandy beaches offered in lieu of a garden.

It seemed like a fair deal: we would accept new technologies, which would modify our habits and oblige us to adjust to certain changes, but in exchange we would be granted relief from the burden of work, more security, and above all, the freedom to pursue our desires. The sacrifice was worth the gain; there would be no regrets. Yet it has become apparent that this civilization of leisure was, in reality, a Trojan horse. Its bulging flanks hid the impositions of a new type of servitude. The automatons are not as autonomous as advertised. They need us. Those computers that were supposed to do our calculations for us instead demand our attention: for ten hours a day, we are glued to their screens. Our communications monopolize our time. Time itself is accelerating. The complexity of the system staggers us. And leisure is often a costly diversion. The beaches, of course, are still there, in high definition on our TV screens.

This is the context in which professional exhaustion appears. Watching pale-faced workers filing from their offices, wrung dry by a system they no longer control, one cannot help but think that they must feel betrayed. Their hopes were high; their disillusionment is bitter. The conditions they endure are familiar to all of us: increasingly powerful production regimes, accelerating rhythms of life, intensification of stress, increasingly invasive instruments of control, and ever-mounting pressure. That is the price we pay for our promised civilization of leisure, which we glimpse mainly through television advertisements.

But this technological expansion is not a spontaneous process. It is driven by an economic logic that seeks, above all, to maximize profits.

In these times of crisis, there is a violence to such logic. In order to compete in a global market, costs must be cut, the workforce must be culled. Mind-blowing systems of management are invented. They subjugate, control, coerce, reward informers and undermine feelings of solidarity. Humans are a resource: they, too, must be made to disgorge their energy, their sweat, their time. Individuals are in all respects supernumerary, and thus replaceable. Consequently, we are experiencing the resurgence of a deep-seated emotion—one that humanism has always sought to expel, and that those in power have often sought to exploit: fear. It is jarring, in this day and age, to look at glistening, glass-plated buildings made of steel, or gleaming robotic assembly lines, and to glimpse beside them workers' faces tense with fear. Surrounded by the trappings of progress, they are the symbols of a regression.

What is burnout, if not a direct result of these excessive regimes? Fatigue, anxiety, unmanageable stress, depersonalization, feelings of incompetence—from this list of symptoms emerges a picture of people who have given too much without getting what they needed, who have neglected their own needs, not always by choice. We will have the opportunity to examine more closely the multifarious nature of this syndrome. Its borders are hazy; its symptoms manifest differently for different people. The contributing factors, equally diverse, can nonetheless be grouped into several broad categories: unsustainable perfectionism, the exhaustion of humanist impulses, the quest for validation, and in addition, the challenges that women, in particular, face.

Rarely does a new psychological disorder capture the attention of the general public so soon after it is first identified. The term was introduced in the 1970s by the American psychiatrist Herbert Freudenberger, who used it to describe his own state of exhaustion in the course of his work with drug addicts at a clinic in New York. It soon came to be used in a variety of contexts, eliciting numerous questions. Is burnout linked to depression? Who are the people most at risk? How can their condition be diagnosed and treated? In seeking the answers to these questions, one is inevitably struck by the humanity of the physicians, psychiatrists, and psychologists who have treated those affected by this syndrome. Their insightful analyses have improved our understanding of the disorder and pointed out paths towards recovery.

In the spirit of their analyses, but from the perspective of a different domain, our aim will be to establish connections between these psychopathological questions and the philosophical inquiries that they give rise to. Our investigation of these inquiries will lead us to reflect on the evocation of fire in the term burnout, which corresponds to a metaphorical conflagration within the individual. We will trace its ancestry, from medieval depictions of acedia, an affliction which prompted monks to lose faith in the divine system, to the British novelist Graham Greene, who first used the term in 1959, on a visit to a leper colony in the Belgian Congo. In the course of our investigation, we will also propose some intentionally outlandish perspectives on this phenomenon, with the goal of inviting further reflection and demonstrating that the problems described are of universal relevance.

Ultimately, it is the institution of work that must be defended. Burnout is not a condition caused by laziness. Those affected are conscientious, passionate, devoted to their work. In fact, that is part of their problem. It would be a grave mistake to reduce the debate to a conflict between activity and idleness. Work is a societal value, a source of emancipation. Its organization is inherently political. It fosters "cooperation," to borrow a term from the psychiatrist Christophe Dejours; it teaches us ways of living together. This is why the egregious abuses that today contribute to its degradation must be viewed as a threat to one of our most basic human needs.

To conclude this introduction, we must highlight what is perhaps the most important aspect of burnout: its potential to bring about metamorphosis. Our bodies are intelligent. They often know more about our needs than do our blinkered psyches. If they beg us for a reprieve, we must listen to them, and let them guide us toward a more viable and fulfilling path. The long-neglected notion of meaning resurfaces with the insistence of a nagging question that cannot be silenced. What is truly important? Where is the center? What is the value of this life?

Emergence from the *nigredo* of burnout is often an excruciating ordeal. But if it can open our minds to these questions, and give us the courage to explore them uncompromisingly, the suffering will not have been in vain.

Confronted with this pathology of post-modern civilization, it is essential that we remain aware of our natural limits as human beings. We cannot tolerate a system that seeks to push beyond those limits in order to more effectively exploit us. In every epoch of history, the proponents of humanism have had to adjust their aims in response to the times. In this day and age, it seems that humanism has one clear task: to once more relegate the logic of economics and technology to a secondary role, so that they may act in the service of goals that are more meaningful, more philosophical, and more humane.

Part I

Beyond Fatigue

Freudenberger and the free clinic

Born in Germany in 1926, Herbert J. Freudenberger came to the United States as a refugee at the age of fifteen. In the 1970s, he worked in one of New York's free clinics, where a largely volunteer staff sought to provide treatment for drug addicts, to prevent overdoses and bad acid trips. However, it quickly became apparent that the addicts weren't the only people at the clinic in need of help. The staff were also showing signs of mental and emotional exhaustion. Freudenberger, a psychiatrist and psychoanalyst, recalled that during this period, he tended to his medical practice at the hospital from 8:00 a.m. to 6:00 p.m., then rushed to the free clinic, working with patients until closing time at 11:00 p.m., after which he would hold staff meetings, returning home around 2:00 a.m. He kept up this routine for months on end. If others suggested that he was working too much, his reply was always the same: "You think I should be doing less? I should be doing more. There are thousands of these kids, and they have no other place to turn." And when people commented that he was getting thinner and thinner, he would reply laconically, "So's Frank Sinatra."[1]

Freudenberger saw himself becoming increasingly cynical and, at times, incapable of responding to his patients' needs. Around him, some of his colleagues were suffering nervous breakdowns, while others abandoned their volunteer work entirely, in spite of their commitment to the cause. At last, he agreed to take some time off for a vacation with his family. The night before their scheduled departure, he returned from

1 H.J. Freudenberger and G. Richardson, *Burn-Out. The High Cost of High Achievement*, London, Arrow Edition, 1985, p. xix (1st ed. New York, Doubleday).

work, as usual, at 2:00 a.m. The following morning, he found himself unable to get out of bed, and the plane left without them. He slept for three days. Upon awakening, he got out his tape recorder and started to talk about his experiences. It was on listening to the resulting tapes that he became fully aware of the change in his personality. He was shocked to hear the strained tone of his own voice, in which he detected exhaustion, anger, depression, arrogance, and when he spoke of his family, guilt. These self-analysis sessions were cathartic for him. Alternating with periods of sleep, they allowed him to regain his footing, to make sense of what had happened to him, and to give a name to his condition.

The term burnout is sometimes used to describe addicts whose excessive drug use has taken its toll on their mental faculties. But little by little, Freudenberger's focus shifted to the mental state of the caregivers, which was not without analogy to that of their patients. The similarity between the symptoms of the patients and those of their caregivers was sufficiently striking, in the view of Freudenberger and his colleagues, that it justified a shift in the application of the word, from one group to the other—an unusual occurrence in the annals of medical history. The term was very quickly adopted by others. Freudenberger began using it with members of his team, and each time, their reaction was one of immediate identification: "Yeah, that's how I feel. Burned out."[2]

The caregivers had been ravaged by forces as toxic as the drugs their patients abused: they were over-worked, perhaps overly idealistic, and certainly over-committed. Like substance abuse, burnout is an illness of immoderation. The intersection of these two worlds is neatly summed up in the construction of the portmanteau word "workaholic." Both conditions are characterized by a disruption of balance. A normal human activity becomes addictive and tyrannically controlling, putting a match to the normal functioning of mental and physical systems. It is

[2] An alternate use of the term is equally evocative: because the tires of drag-racing vehicles perform better at higher temperatures, drivers at the starting line of a race may set their tires spinning at maximum torque while simultaneously engaging the brake. During a burnout, the car remains stationary, but the engine revs at full throttle, releasing smoke. This image can be readily transposed to a psychological context: the individual reaches maximum exertion but cannot move forward.

no coincidence that the term "burnout" suggests the aftermath of a fire. For Freudenberger, the metaphor of fire is deeply evocative:

> As a practicing psychoanalyst, I have come to realize that people, as well as buildings, sometimes burn out. Under the strain of living in our complex world, their inner resources are consumed as if by fire, leaving a great emptiness inside, although their outer shells may be more or less unchanged.[3]

Fatigue is an intrinsic counterpart to human activity. Every human exertion requires power, energy combustion, hormonal regulation, increased blood circulation and pulmonary respiration. When the limits of these somatic functions are exceeded, subjective manifestations up to and including total exhaustion inevitably result.[4] Nonetheless, while burnout may be accompanied by the symptoms of normal physical exhaustion, the fatigue associated with burnout has its own particular qualities. It is not at all like the fatigue of workers performing strenuous physical labor, nor does it resemble the wild-eyed, tormented sleeplessness experienced by soldiers engaged in trench warfare, Nazi officers deprived of amphetamines, or American soldiers in Iraq. It is not comparable to the kind of fatigue that keeps night-shift workers rubbing their eyes, nor to the type of prolonged sleep deprivation that results in short-term memory impairment. It has almost nothing in common with the exertions of elite athletes, nor is it comparable to the intellectual fatigue of compulsive readers or of scientists who single-mindedly pursue a line of inquiry. And it is emphatically not the sluggishness that results from inactivity.

A weariness rooted in the will to succeed, to work diligently and go the extra mile, even if it means neglecting one's own, basic needs, the fatigue of burnout is often downplayed by the sufferer, perceived as an obstacle to productivity. The signal gets lost amidst the noise of so many other imperatives and exigencies. It persists as a dull, nagging tiredness: an omnipresent feeling of deficiency which the sufferer tries to silence,

3 Freudenberger, *Burn-Out. The High Cost of High Achievement*, *op. cit.*, p. xv.

4 J. Scherrer, *La Fatigue*. Paris, PUF, 1989, p. 101.

as if giving the body a chance to catch its breath would be an admission of weakness. Victims of burnout may turn to drugs to mask the exhaustion responsible for this shameful incapacity. By this stage, they can no longer deal with conflicts, or else they provoke them outrageously, but are helpless to resolve them. They become more and more isolated, believing that alone, they will be better able to mediate the conflict between one part of themselves that begs for a reprieve and another that demands one more effort, one more burst of energy. In this way, the individual begins to split in two. This phenomenon may be exteriorized in various different ways: for some, it manifests as sarcasm, irony, cynicism, or a feeling of invincibility; for others, it results in binge eating, excessive drinking, or exaggerated sexuality. But in each case, the self divided by an internal struggle is driven toward destruction and transformation. The victim's behavior changes noticeably; people close to her begin to worry. The gulf widens between the yearning for repose and the drive to keep going at all costs, motivated by supposedly sound reasons—financial gain, social status, professional success—until at last it consumes the individual. Torn in two by this internal schism, she becomes "depersonalized."[5] She loses touch with herself and her own needs. Her field of view is limited to the present time, which is divided up into a series of mechanical tasks to be completed. Fatigue, which for so long had been kept at bay, now becomes untamable. No amount of willpower can hold it in check. It spreads out, engulfing the victim's entire being, physical, emotional, and intellectual. It is at this point that the metaphor of burning comes fully into play: the victim feels an emptiness spreading inside her, as fast-moving as a wildfire, as inexorable as flame. She becomes that emptiness, that scorched landscape.

Christina Maslach, professor of psychology at the University of California at Berkeley and creator of the "Maslach Burnout Inventory," a test used worldwide to assess symptoms of burnout, has demonstrated that this process actually involves three different dimensions, which do not always coincide. First, and most visible, is the dimension of

5 Ulrich Kraft, "Burned Out," *Scientific American Mind*, June–July 2006, pp. 28–33.

exhaustion, the body's primary reaction to long-term exposure to stress. The individual feels "drained, used up, and unable to unwind or recover."[6] Next is the dimension of depersonalization, most often signaled by the voicing of cynical pronouncements. Freudenberger himself commented on the significance of this cynicism. Those afflicted by burnout prefer to maintain a cold and distant attitude toward their colleagues and show less devotion to their jobs. Their cynicism is protective; their negativity proclaims that they have no more illusions about the value of their work. The third dimension of burnout, according to Maslach, is that of inefficacity: each new project feels overwhelming, prompting the individual to lose confidence.

Maslach's work is also notable for the fact that she explicitly addresses the ways in which social environment contributes to burnout. For her, and for the majority of psychologists, it is impossible to account for this disorder by attributing it solely to some deficiency in the individual sufferer. Her convictions are clearly expressed in the following declaration:

> Burnout is reaching epidemic proportions among North American workers today. It's not so much that something has gone wrong with us but rather that there have been fundamental changes in the workplace and the nature of our jobs. The workplace today is a cold, hostile, demanding environment, both economically and psychologically. People are emotionally, physically, and spiritually exhausted. The daily demands of the job, the family, and everything in between erode their energy and enthusiasm. The joy of success and the thrill of achievement are more and more difficult to attain. Dedication and commitment to the job are fading. People are becoming cynical, keeping their distance, trying not to let themselves get too involved.[7]

At this point, no one could dispute the social dimension of burnout. It is not simply a psychological failing of the individual: the type, quantity, and difficulty of the work, lack of control, perceptions of unfairness,

[6] C. Maslach and M. Leiter, *The Truth about Burnout*. San Francisco, Wiley, 1997, p. 17.

[7] *Ibid.*, p. 1.

insufficient rewards, and interpersonal conflicts are also implicated, in varying proportions. Freudenberger would never have asserted otherwise. Burnout, for him, was the affliction of the "good American," whose dreams are aligned with the dominant values of work, money, ingenuity, discovery, industrialization, self-improvement, and finally, the imposition of democratic values, including liberty and free enterprise, on the rest of the world. It afflicts those who are most faithful to the system, the "true believers." It is their crisis of faith: the disillusionment of the dreamers, the exhaustion of those who gave their utmost to the construction of this society, and who had expected to blossom under its auspices. This aspect of burnout has implications that go beyond, and also complement, the insights offered by psychology and sociology. Burnout replaces the richness of a healthy relationship between individuals and their work with an immense void of meaninglessness. What is lost is not just the ability to work or the capacity to derive satisfaction from one's efforts. The meaning of the activity is itself destroyed, reduced to nothing. This loss has a signification that merits closer examination, for clearly it extends beyond the experience of individual sufferers. Burnout refers to a type of exhaustion, but it has many other dimensions. If we are to bring them all to light, we must begin by exploring the true origins of the concept.

Tired souls

Burnout has a long-forgotten ancestor, with characteristics that give us additional insight into this complex problem. The symptoms were described as follows: "Physical exhaustion, fatigue, hunger, increased frequency or intensity of temptations, prolonged absence of sensible consolations, bitterness resulting from real or apparent failures in the struggle against evil or from reprimands, whether deserved or undeserved; the simple monotony of daily routines and the need for change that we all naturally experience may be at the root of this crisis ..." But for a few minor details, this could be mistaken for an excerpt from a pamphlet on burnout or a self-help book. Two words that seem incongruous with modern terminology are "temptations" and "reprimands." In the jargon of today's business consultants—a sort of plutocratic Newspeak—the equivalents might be "I've removed him from my LinkedIn contacts" or "We're putting her on a performance improvement plan."[8] Equally obsolete, and more incendiary, is "evil," a four-letter word that no one today would dare to use. But, setting aside these semantic reservations, the description remains applicable.

It is, in fact, an excerpt from a dictionary of Catholic theology published in 1932. In the entry concerning "sloth," we find an important reflection on acedia that gives us every reason to view it as an ancient form of burnout. Acedia was for the Church what burnout has become for the business world: a dreaded affliction that incapacitates the individual, but also, more threateningly, undermines his faith in the system. This explains why it is taken so seriously. Acedia is qualitatively different from other forms of sloth. It is distinct from the more run-of-the-mill variety known as *pigritia*, an avoidance of effort which the Church considers sinful. An exaggerated love of comfort and leisure distances the believer from God and duty. It challenges the terrible order of Genesis, "by the sweat of your brow you will eat bread until you return to the ground" and shrugs off Pascal's fretful pronouncement that "there must be no sleep while Christ is in agony." Inevitably, it becomes a sensual trap: the idler, grown weary, will soon take to his bed, alone or alongside his equally idle consort. To cure him of his vice, medieval tracts proposed putting him to work, showing him a field covered with brambles and thorns, or a broken-down wall in need of repair.[9] There is no indication as to the effectiveness of this treatment,

8 For more examples (in French) of this Newspeak, see the glossary of the excellent and tragic book by Alexandre des Isnards and Thomas Zuber, *L'open space m'a tuer* [*Open space killd me*] (*sic*), which "describes everything that all young executives know but won't tell anyone else: the newest forms of violence, the diktat of good humor and conviviality, the false freedom of flextime, the torment of the timesheet, the folly of employee assessment and self-evaluation, the lack of recognition, etc.": Paris, Le Livre de Poche, 2008, p. 13.

9 *Dictionnaire de théologie catholique* [*Dictionary of Catholic Theology*], article on "Paresse [Sloth]," by E. Vansteenberghe, Letouzey Ed., 1932, Vol. XI, part 2.

but the Church does not seem to have made the success of the cure a priority.

Acedia, in contrast, was regarded as a genuine threat, for it was a form of sloth directed at God. It would strike unexpectedly, afflicting those monks who were most fastidious in their faith, most methodical in their duties and diligent in their daily prayers, who ordinarily would never shirk from a supplementary fast or an additional early morning service. Yet, from time to time, these monks would break down. Acedia was a monastic version of burnout, affecting the monk's spiritual life and his relationship with God, just as modern burnout transforms the worker's professional life and her relationship to her company. In the eleventh century, Guigo I described it as follows:

> Often, alone in your cell, you are seized by a sort of inertia, a spiritual languor, an ennui of the heart, and so you feel within you an unbearable sense of disgust: you are a burden to yourself; those internal graces, which you used to draw upon so joyfully, no longer hold for you any sweetness; the tenderness that was in you yesterday and the day before has been transformed into a great bitterness.[10]

The Desert Fathers, Cassian, Saint John Climacus, Isidore of Seville, Saint Thomas, and many others devoted considerable attention to acedia, due to its frequency of occurrence among hermits and in monasteries. It should be emphasized that acedia often took hold of the most promising monks, the most fervent practitioners of their religion. Monks who had never doubted, who seemed to be on their way to sainthood, one day found themselves tired of God. For that is precisely what they were experiencing: spiritual fatigue. Soon, the Our Fathers just wouldn't come; the sufferer would genuflect and find he had no strength to rise. Then came the forgotten Ave Marias and, in the middle of the morning service, a diabolical urge to sleep. Saint John Cassian, quoted by Jean-Louis Chrétien in his very beautiful book on fatigue, devoted an entire section of his *Institutes of the Coenobia* to acedia, which he defined as *tædium sive anxietas cordis*, "tedium or anxiety of

[10] *Ibid.*, p. 2026.

the heart." According to Cassian, the monk experiences "such bodily weariness and longing for food that he seems to himself worn out and wearied as if with a long journey, or some very heavy work, or as if he had put off taking food during a fast of two or three days ... and so a kind of unreasonable confusion of mind takes possession of him like some foul darkness, and makes him idle and useless for every spiritual work, so that he imagines that no cure for so terrible an attack can be found in anything except visiting some one of the brethren, or in the solace of sleep alone."[11]

Acedia is a cardinal sin. Saint John Climacus regards it as one of the gravest of vices, since it attacks the source of all virtue, rather than one virtue in particular. To be tired of God, and ultimately to reject the divine good, is to deny oneself any possibility of redemption. In the eyes of the theologians, there is nothing more pernicious. It would be like losing interest in one's job in a society that fetishizes work... No wonder the theologians sought remedies for this spiritual affliction turned sin, just as today's managers call for solutions to the scourge of burnout. The remedy proposed by the theologians was to think of death and of future rewards, in order to re-awaken hope and courage. They also counselled perseverance, advising the afflicted "to hold firm, abandoning neither their state in life, nor their abbey, nor their duties; ... to act through study, chanting, physical labor, prayer, and all manner of good works."[12]

At the same time, work remained an object of suspicion. The Franciscan theologian Bernard Forthomme, in an impressive volume devoted to the subject, speaks of "acedia as overwork." He analyzes examples of what the ancients called "the demon of work" to show that the Fathers of the Church considered acedia a disease of excess, not of idleness. It is the excess of prayer that overwhelms faith. The "evil spirit" incites the desire to always be doing more. It urges the religious devotee

11 *The Twelve Books of John Cassian on the Institutes of the Coenobia, and the Remedies for the Eight Principal Faults.* Translated by Edgar C.S. Gibson, from *A Select Library of Nicene and Post-Nicene Fathers of the Christian Church, Second Series, Vol. 11.* New York, 1894. (Quoted in French in Jean-Louis Chrétien's *De la fatigue* [*On Fatigue*], Paris, Minuit, 1996, p. 94.)

12 *Dictionnaire de théologie catholique, op. cit.*, Vol. XI, part 2, p. 2030.

to construct four or five cells, when one or two would suffice. "The friar overcome with fatigue wishes to rest, to put an end to his work. But the evil spirit excites and animates him, never letting go. There is no release. He must keep his hammer in hand … *indefatigable*."[13] Acedia stems from an excess of work, which is another way in which it parallels the condition that Freudenberger labeled burnout.

An interesting distinction nonetheless separates these two afflictions. Acedia was seen as a "cooling down." The word acedia was associated with the Latin *acidus*, because acidic things were believed to be cooling. Fervor, which is associated with fire and heat, gives way to what theologians called "tepidness" of the soul, which "neutralizes completely the fervent commitment to charity, the flame that burns ardently."[14] From this perspective, burnout and acedia could be seen as opposites. Catholic theology, which valorizes fervor and enthusiasm, repudiates the kind of cold, dispassionate reasoning that could lead to atheism. In contrast, technological systems, built on cold logic, are wary of excessive zealousness, suspecting perhaps that it gives rise to conflict.

Burnout is an acedia for our times. The similarities are striking. But most striking of all is the fact that these two afflictions lead to the same outcome: a loss of faith. The Church, in its role as a religious enterprise, perceived acedia as a serious threat, because it led monks to doubt the existence of God. There could be nothing worse. In the same way, burnout has a devastating effect on modern businesses because it calls into question the values they represent. The omnipresence of stress is perceived as an attempt at manipulation. Work ethic, which had been the motor of activity, disappears. Motivation erodes. Like the monk who can no longer bear to pray to a God who no longer comforts him, the worker throws up her hands, often in response to a lack of

13 Bernard Forthomme, *De l'acédie monastique à l'anxio-dépression. Histoire philosophique de la transformation d'un vice en pathologie* [*From Monastic Acedia to Anxiety and Depression: a Philosophical History of the Transformation of a Vice into a Pathology*], Paris, Les empêcheurs de penser en rond, 2000, p. 31.

14 *Dictionnaire de théologie catholique*, *op. cit.*, Vol. XV, part 1, article on "Tiédeur [Tepidness]," p. 1026. See also Forthomme's *De l'acédie monastique*, op. cit.: "L'indévotion comme tiédeur [Lack of Devotion as Tepidness]," p. 418.

recognition. She begins to have doubts. She asks herself if the purpose of her brief existence could possibly be wholehearted devotion to a multinational company that doesn't know she exists, to shareholders who look upon her with indifference. She has lost faith in herself, but above all, she has lost faith in a system that seems to treat her with contempt. Her faith in herself will, hopefully, return. But her belief in the system has been permanently shaken. Burnout always calls into question the dominant system of values: it produces new non-believers who can no longer worship at the altar of techno-capitalism.

In a Congolese leper colony

In addition to exhaustion and loss of faith, there is another element embedded in the history of the word burnout. Poets and writers often act as prospectors for the social sciences. They bring to the surface ideas in their native state, as yet unmarked by interpretation, but closely linked to a particular context and environment. They mine human experience so that others may analyze it. Through an imaginative transformation of observed experience, they uncover singular truths, bringing them to the attention of more intellectually rigorous disciplines. The case of burnout is a telling example. Freudenberger, as we have seen, was the first to provide a systematic description of this notion, giving it a coherent meaning in the context of the social sciences. But he was neither the originator of the term nor the concept. The demiurge truly responsible for their genesis was the British novelist Graham Greene, who in 1961 published *A Burnt-Out Case*, a novel that undoubtedly found its way onto Freudenberger's night table.

The novel's chilling epigraph, borrowed from Dante, sets the tone for the narrative that follows: *Io non mori, e non rimasi vivo.* "I did not die, yet nothing of life remained." This laconic statement describes the mental landscape of Querry, an internationally renowned architect whom life has seemingly favored. Irresistible to women, rich, perhaps even handsome in his youth, he finds himself, at the end of yet another romantic entanglement, embarking from an airport in Belgium for the former colony of Congo. When we first encounter him, he is in the midst of a two-week journey up a river in an old boat, which takes him, when the road and the river have reached their end and there is truly no further means to flee, to a leper colony. It is here that Querry sets down his baggage, literally and figuratively. No one asks anything of him. At first, he is a mere observer, insisting that nothing interests him. "I've come through to the other side, to nothing."[15] But in this nothing, Querry finds a possibility of life. The lepers suffer; the Belgian priests and an atheist doctor attempt to relieve their suffering. Querry is transformed. But in what way? As a writer, Greene is neither naïve enough to equate proximity to death with redemption, nor Catholic enough to turn his novel into an allegory in which God is glimpsed in the disfigured faces of the lepers. His focus is on a different type of revelation. He imagines a psychological transformation of a type never before described.

Greene had, of course, been to Africa himself. The novel draws on his own experiences. The observations he recorded in his notebooks, published under the title *In Search of a Character*, offer valuable insight into his writing process. The reader can follow him, plotting the path his hero would later take through the Belgian Congo, up a river and into a leper colony, obsessed, like any other professional novelist, with the creation of a believable character. He had the idea of a man who has "come to the end of his vocation." As he wrote in his journal, "the love of his art has gone the way of his love of women: a kind of sensual exhaustion has overtaken that too."[16] This character would, naturally, develop into Querry. A bit further on in his notes, in an entry dated February 10, 1959, we find the following words, which amount to a birth announcement for an idea:

> Leprosy cases whose disease has been arrested and cured only after the loss of fingers and toes are known as burnt-out cases. This is the parallel

[15] Graham Greene, *A Burnt-Out Case*, New York, Viking Press, 1961, p. 90.
[16] Graham Greene, *In Search of a Character: Two African Journals*. New York, Viking Press, 1961, p. 16.

> I have been seeking between my character X and the lepers. Psychologically and morally he has been burnt-out. Is it at that point that the cure is effected?[17]

Like Freudenberger, Greene turns to metaphors. Freudenberger described his drug-addicted patients as "burnt out" before applying the description to his own condition. For his part, Greene borrowed a term from the medical treatment of leprosy to characterize the mental state of his hero. From the addict to the doctor, from the leper to the hero, these metaphors follow a parallel course and, in both cases, serve as tools for comprehension. Metaphors are never gratuitous. A basic structure of our language and of our psychological universe, they are more than a matter of words. Metaphors are an intrinsic element of "human *thought processes*,"[18] an effort to understand the invisible by means of the visible, the unknown by means of the known. In this instance, the unknown is a mental disorder. Before burnout, other psychological conditions had already been assigned significations by means of metaphors. Thus hysteria, which evokes the displacement of the uterus, and depression, which connotes concavity, both make reference to physical experience—however inaccurately, in the case of hysteria—in order to describe a state of mind.[19]

17 *Ibid.*, p. 26. Greene includes an important footnote: "The English phrase is used by the Belgian doctors—there is no French equivalent, and for that reason I had to find quite a different title for my novel in French." This title, *La Saison des pluies* [*Rainy Season*], is decidedly more prosaic than the original, although it does evoke the relief that comes when the intense African heat gives way to cooling rains. It remains the earliest testimony to the untranslatability of the term "burnout." The doctor who inspired the book was Baron Michel Lechat (1927–2014).

18 G. Lakoff and M. Johnson, *Metaphors We Live By*, Chicago, University of Chicago Press, 1980, p. 6. Emphasis in original.

19 The writer William Styron is one of those who object to the inadequate and "bland" metaphor on which the word depression is constructed, to the point of requesting that a different, more arresting metaphor, like "tempest in the brain," be used in its place. "'Melancholia,'" he writes, "would still appear to be a far more apt and evocative word for the blacker forms of the disorder, but it was usurped by a noun with a blank tonality and lacking any magisterial presence, used indifferently to describe an economic decline or a rut in the ground, a true wimp of a word for such a major illness" (William Styron, *Darkness Visible: A Memoir of Madness*. New York, Random House, 1990, p. 37). In comparison, the metaphor of "burnout" is actually more explicit.

If metaphors are not gratuitous, neither are they innocuous. Intellectual lines of descent sometimes take surprising turns, and words, like arrows flying in fractal formation, keep the imprint of the bow that launched them. In this instance, there is a certain irony to the fact that an affliction now rampant in the world of techno-capitalism owes its name to a condition suffered by lepers, exiled and ostracized from every society in every part of the world. There is something biblical in this association between words, justified, according to Greene, by an analogy between the two afflictions. It creates a strange intimacy between the powerful and the downtrodden, in parallel states of vulnerability.

We are left with the question of what it was that leprosy allowed Greene to understand about his protagonist. Querry has been lauded as a visionary architect, but he has no more delusions of grandeur. He sees the limitations of his talent. He knows that vanity and money were his motivation, and that, compared to the work of the architects who constructed Chartres, inspired by love and faith, the "box of concrete and glass (he) landed on a poor city square"[20] is an ugly and grotesque edifice. His work has become absurd to him. Neither fame nor accolades can fill the void. He feels he has reached the end of his talent. Greene presents a parable to illustrate this realization. He compares his protagonist to a skilled jeweler who fashions a jewel in the form of an ostrich egg: "it was all enamel and gold and when you opened it you found inside a little gold figure sitting at a table and a little gold-and-enamel egg on the table, and when you opened that there was a little figure sitting at a table, and when you opened that there was a little figure sitting at a table and a little gold-and-enamel egg . . ."[21] In these nested boxes carved with increasingly miniscule representations of their creator, Querry's alter ego is confronted by a revelation: he has arrived at the end of pleasure, the end of his profession. One day, gazing into the egg, he feels nothing but boredom. The ingeniousness of his work as a jeweler has worn him out. And, certainly, when life resembles

[20] Graham Greene, *A Burnt-Out Case*, New York, Viking Press, 1961. *op. cit.*, p. 138.
[21] *Ibid.*, p. 193.

a succession of Russian dolls, when the point of existence diminishes and grows narrower with each passing day, lassitude threatens.

For Querry, it is the same with women. An inveterate seducer, he no longer feels love. As with any insatiable Don Juan, undressing a woman arouses his desire not for her naked body, but for the next undressing. The body of one woman anticipates the clothing of another, whose nudity in turn becomes a prelude to the next conquest. This succession of lovers is imbricated in his fantasies like a series of nested boxes. Each fleeting gratification reignites his desire, in a cycle of futile frivolity, the reality of which is expressed in Nerval's famous verse: "The thirteenth returns, and is again the first . . ." Until one morning, this rondo reveals itself to be a vain and tedious dance. It becomes a caricature of its own absurd repetition, always ending in ennui. It was on such a morning, undoubtedly, that Querry embarked for Africa.

In modern parlance, we would call this a classic case of burnout. In urgent need of treatment. But Greene would say otherwise. He does not use the expression "burnt-out" to describe the lost and exhausted man boarding a plane to a randomly selected destination, certain that what awaits him can be no worse than what he leaves behind. This man is depressed, weary to the point of muteness, but he is not yet burnt out, contrary to our current usage of the term. For Greene, "burnt-out" refers to the recovery phase. The text is clear: for the inventor of this metaphor, it is only when Querry has reached the end of his process of disillusionment and the combustion of everything within him that had become false and infected, only when he has completely burned through his self-contempt, that he will be "burnt-out." Burnout is what comes after the illness, the beginning of renewal. This may come as a surprise to us, but it makes sense if we return to the analogy with leprosy that guides the author's construction. In the novel, the doctor uses this term to refer to lepers who are no longer "infectious."[22] The virulent phases of this devastating disease are characterized by damage and loss of sensation in the nerve cells, leading to loss of limbs, disfigurement, or

[22] *Ibid.*, p. 135.

mutilation. The horrific lesions that scar the skin result from these attacks on the nerve endings which, after manifesting violently, may subside. At this point, the disease is said to have run its course, to have "burnt out." The patient is a "burnt-out case." He has lost, "everything that can be eaten away before (being) cured."[23] To say that such patients are now healed would be inaccurate, since they will always carry the scars and the stigma of leprosy in their disfigurement. But they are no longer contagious. *Consummatum est*. It is finished, or, as an alternate rendering of the Latin might have it: all has been consumed.

Such is the clinical presentation of one of the most degrading illnesses in existence. It was this set of symptoms that Graham Greene contemplated and transposed to the psychological and moral state of his protagonist. When he arrives in Africa, Querry is still full of infection: self-hatred, disgust, lassitude, ambivalence about his own success, self-deception and, above all, fear. "I am afraid to return,"[24] he remarks. We can see that his problem is also of a "moral" order. His time in the leper colony with the patients, the doctor and the priests, has the effect of burning away all of his fears, all the distorted ideas and neuroses that the pursuit of success has brought him. He is consumed and stripped bare. The "old man" within him, who fed on success, vanity and wealth, dies, as does the fantasy of finding meaning in an existence built on lies, infidelity, and puerile narcissism. It is a catharsis, a cleansing, a liberation. Recognizing that "(s)uccess is . . . a mutilation of the natural man,"[25] Querry strips himself of it. This self-immolation brings him to a point where he can say: "*Consummatum est*: pain over and peace falling round . . . like a little death."[26]

Did Greene himself experience an episode of this type? Is he writing from personal experience? It is difficult to say. A reading of his journal shows him to be concerned above all with the credibility of his character and the singularity of his experience. The shadow of Joseph Conrad

[23] *Ibid*., pp. 18 and 132.
[24] *Ibid*., p. 28.
[25] *Ibid*., p. 245.
[26] *Ibid*., p. 152.

hovers over Greene's story, since, like Marlowe in *Heart of Darkness*, Querry journeys up an African river that will lead him toward the dark and mysterious reaches of human experience. Certainly, Conrad's style is more expansive, profound and subtle than that of Greene, who is more concerned with expediency. Still, both authors share the ability to unfurl their imaginations against a stark background and transform it in the service of an aesthetic, intellectual and moral generosity that gives their work a greater sense of purpose and meaning. Such was Conrad's mission, as Jean-Jacques Mayoux explains in his introduction to the French edition of *Heart of Darkness*: "With his prodigious imagination, to break through the walls of solitude that enclose people externally and separate them internally from their deepest essence; to bear witness, to reveal, to serve as a vicarious, sympathetic consciousness for those who could not know themselves or one another."[27] Greene is working in the same modality, in search of the word that will imbue his fictional characters with a coherence that ordinary human beings, lost in their own complexity, rarely possess. The peculiar thing is that, today, this word is more often heard in business back rooms than at the bedsides of lepers.

"I think I'm cured of pretty well everything, even disgust. I've been happy here":[28] these are Querry's last words before his senseless death at the hands of a jealous husband whose wife had invented a non-existent liaison between herself and Querry as a premise for escaping Africa and an unhappy marriage. A sad death for a man who had made the effort to see one of his lives through to its end, only to succumb on the brink of a metamorphosis. But these last words resonate like Dante's glorious "*Incipit vita nova*." He has returned from hell. Everything has burned, but he remains. And for those of us who find in them the kernel of an idea, those final words: "I've been happy here," the culmination of this episode of personal transformation, sound like an unexpected truth. This does not mean that we should conceive of burnout as a desirable

[27] J.-J. Mayoux, Introduction to the French edition of J. Conrad, *Heart of Darkness* [*Au coeur des ténèbres*], Paris, Flammarion, 1989, p. 33.

[28] Graham Greene, *A Burnt-Out Case*, New York, Viking Press, 1961. *op. cit.*, p. 241.

condition; that would be an over-romanticization. But it does indicate that the shedding of certain contemporary fantasies that haunt our brains is not always a source of unhappiness. Burnout, from its inception, has been suffused with considerable ambiguity.

Taken in its native state, burnout signifies a type of metamorphosis that leads to a catharsis. The individual enters into battle against the illusions, beliefs, and dominant values to which she can no longer claim allegiance and ultimately sloughs them off. This universal theme has always guided those who sought to be reborn into a more authentic existence: philosophers, seekers, religious initiates, mystics, all those who follow a path of transformation. The notion of burnout carries with it the same moral and philosophical weight, which is the source of its underlying duality.

Exhaustion, loss of faith, and then, hopefully, metamorphosis: from the beginning, the significance of burnout has extended beyond the sphere of psychology. What appears to be a struggle with oneself or against a frustrating environment culminates in the indictment of an entire society. It will become apparent, as we examine the factors in today's working world that can lead to this disorder, that they also extend beyond the dimension of the individual. They concern civilization in its entirety.

Part II

The Burnout Machine

Abandoning perfection

The job that Matthew B. Crawford landed after finishing his degree in philosophy seemed like a perfect fit. It involved reading scientific articles published in specialized magazines and writing abstracts, which would be added to a subscription-only online database. Crawford was intelligent and inquisitive; he liked to write. He was being asked to peruse the prose of geneticists, climatologists, and linguists. The assignment coincided with his aspirations. He was to become a knowledge worker—an attractive prospect in itself, and one that promised a decent salary. His first day on the job in Foster City—a planned community adjacent to Silicon Valley—began with a general orientation.

He quickly learned that he would have to produce fifteen abstracts per day. This quota would oblige him to devote no more than one half-hour to each article, despite his inclinations to give them a more attentive reading. The principles by which the company operated were designed to eliminate any waste of time. Employees were to abide by the golden rule that it is unnecessary to understand the content of an article in order to produce a satisfactory abstract: it would be sufficient to extract the relevant key words and main ideas and assemble them into a few grammatically correct sentences. The resulting product would be accurate enough to keep database users satisfied, or at least, to keep them reaching for their credit cards. Crawford needed a job. He sensed from that first day that the work would be demanding, that it would frustrate him to merely skim through articles that genuinely interested him. He realized, moreover, that he would feel as though he was betraying the authors whose work he summarized, and that he would experience this failure to do justice to their ideas as an act of violence against himself. He perceived all this on his first day, with the kind of unerring intuition that is nonetheless easily disregarded. After all, the pay was good, and he was young and adaptable. It wasn't as if he'd been expecting a sinecure.

All of his apprehensions were confirmed, and then some. After eleven months, his quota had risen to twenty-eight abstracts per day. Articles on rheumatology, fluid mechanics, and sexology flew past him so quickly that he could scarcely distinguish one topic from another, and all the abstracts began to sound the same. The knowledge worker had been reduced to ignorant drudgery. Urged to work at an ever-accelerating pace, he felt like a distant cousin of Charlie Chaplin's character in *Modern Times*, minus the slapstick comedy. His was a mental assembly line, a chaos of key words, a succession of meaningless phrases. Nor was there anyone on hand to verify the accuracy of the abstracts he produced. All that mattered were the quotas, dictated by ambitious managers on the orders of investors who knew nothing whatsoever about the abstractors' work. The symptoms of boredom, fatigue, detachment, cynicism and depression manifested in rapid succession. It's not hard to guess what happened next.

But what happened next had consequences of its own, consequences that ultimately led to the writing of a book—an honorable outcome, as Mallarmé taught us.[1] Crawford had the courage to give up his office job and, eventually, to open a motorcycle repair shop in Virginia. Surrounded by metal, motors, and the tangible problems posed by technical objects, he at last found work that, for him, had inherent meaning and value. In his book *Shop Class as Soulcraft*, he dissects, with unsparing lucidity, the false promises of the knowledge economy. His rehabilitation of manual labor dismantles the unjustifiable superiority complex of white collar workers who never get their hands dirty, whom Crawford describes variously as "estranged labor" and

1 Translator's note: In *Divagations*, published in 1897, Stéphane Mallarmé famously wrote, "Tout, au monde, existe pour aboutir à un livre." ("Everything in the world exists to end up in a book.")

"walking wounded."[2] Having found satisfaction and serenity through hands-on mechanical labor, Crawford talks about technical craft in a manner that unmistakably aligns him with the singular perspective of the philosopher of technology Gilbert Simondon, though there is no indication that he is familiar with Simondon's work.[3] The political and economic ramifications of Crawford's analysis must be carefully considered. It is easy enough to move a call center, or even a revenue office, overseas, but it is impossible to hire a long-distance plumber. You can't hammer in a nail online, as Crawford points out. The limits of globalization reside in our concrete relationship with the world.

Crawford's experience is of particular interest, because in shining a light on the conditions that lead to burnout, it puts to rest two common misconceptions. First, it demonstrates that professional exhaustion does not primarily afflict reluctant workers, but rather those who want to be fully engaged. Contrary to the assertions of many a treatise on idleness,[4] the kind of eagerness to work that Crawford initially manifested is a sentiment many workers feel on a visceral level. The desire to work is often a fundamental drive. This is why unemployment can be such a crushing experience. As Christophe Dejours observes in his analysis of the psychodynamics of work:

> The subjective inclination toward work is strongly manifested in the majority of healthy subjects. It is as if, confronted with the elements of

2 Matthew B. Crawford, *Shop Class as Soulcraft: An Inquiry into the Value of Work*, New York, Penguin Press, 2009, pp. 142–143.

3 Although Crawford arrived at his conclusions independently, he is spiritually indebted to the philosophy of Gilbert Simondon (1924–1989) which calls upon us to consider our relationships with technology and individuation in a new light. Simondon is the spiritual father of all those who, like Crawford, have sought to provide a critical counterpoint to a certain kind of rabidly techno-capitalistic worldview, without adopting a pseudo-humanistic standpoint that places all the blame on technology itself. The importance of this philosophical approach for contemporary thought is further delineated in the postface of this book. See also P. Chabot, *The Philosophy of Simondon*, London, Bloomsbury, 2013, translated by Graeme Krikpatrick and Aliza Krefetz.

4 The authors of these treatises are themselves among the least indolent of all workers, as attested to by their finely honed prose and carefully laid-out propositions. It may be that writing does not feel like work to them, as is the case with any true passion. But it must be conceded, nonetheless, that spending all morning hunched over a desk is an occupation unworthy of a true idler, who will always prefer the shade of the nearest tree.

work, subjects could not help but engage with them, drawing upon all of their intellectual and emotional resources.[5]

The second popular misconception holds that those who are exhausted by work are simply maladapted. In medical write-ups, burnout is sometimes described as "trouble adapting." The expression is as ambiguous as it is surprising. Was the talented Crawford poorly adapted to the task assigned to him? Too stupid or lazy? Or was it the work itself that led to problems of adaptation? On reflection, this debate is formulated around an ideological perspective typical of our current system, which posits that some people are well-adapted while others fail to adapt. This is, however, a flawed premise. In reality, human beings are the most adaptable of all animals. Flexible, resilient, and malleable, we are quick to adjust to novel situations, often deliberately seeking them out. The multitude of adaptive strategies that humans have employed in order to survive and thrive are on display in any ethnological museum. Television, itself a sort of ethnological museum updated in real time, provides ample evidence of our species' capacity to endlessly modify itself and its environment. Every program, every series, is a showcase for the strategies humans use to adapt to complex environments and to get other humans to adapt their behavior in a way that aligns with their desires. But such adaptation is insufficient: we also crave self-realization, the pursuit of a higher goal or purpose. Adaptation is rarely an end in itself, and this is the crux of the problem faced by contemporary society.

The focus on adaptation is a flaw in the dominant ideology. We are informed that people must adapt to their jobs, that employees must conform to company culture, that artists must submit to the codes set in place by cultural industries, that immigrants must assimilate to the values of their adoptive countries. Yet, this approach overlooks the fact that adaptation is often a secondary consideration. It is a means in service of a greater goal, a step towards self-realization, a way of making an impact on the world. We adapt to an environment, but we also

[5] Christophe Dejours, *Travail vivant. 2. Travail et emancipation* [*Work and Emancipation*], Paris, Payot, 2009, p. 103.

attempt to shape it, making modifications that suit our own needs. "To adapt to the world," writes Joseph Nuttin, "is to succeed in adapting the world to oneself."[6] Contrary to conventional wisdom, we do not limit our desires to conform with our current reality. Life is too short to be wholly shaped by the demands of an environment. Even unconsciously, we are driven to transform and restructure our surroundings. Again, in Joseph Nuttin's words: "Everywhere, adaptation is the strategy employed by an organism in order to realize its own structures, by one means or another, within the limits of its environment and its own plasticity."[7] The environment, which is resistant at first, often winds up playing a positive role in this operation. The demands it places on the individual—for example, the economic imperative to work—may in turn give individuals the opportunity to realize their potential.

Burnout is the reflection of an adaptation that has been reduced to frustrating absurdity, because it has become an end in itself. It is the trap set by an impossible perfectionism. The story of Crawford and his abstracts can be read as one man's well-meaning effort to adapt to a set of constraints which, just as they begin to seem bearable, keep recalibrating to become ever more impossible. In this case, the company's management had ensured that workers would never be given time to breathe, using every sign of adaptation as an excuse to present them with "new challenges," which were, in reality, tantamount to harassment.[8] Were it not so tragic, we could compare this work environment to a perverse psychology experiment designed to study the limits of human

6 Joseph Nuttin, "Adaptation," in *Encyclopédie Universalis*, Paris, 1990, volume 1, p. 256. Nuttin's excellent article on adaptation has been replaced in more recent editions by an entry less focused on these questions.

7 *Ibid.* In *L'Individuation psychique et collective* [*Psychic and Collective Individuation*] (Paris, Aubier, 1989), Gilbert Simondon pursues the same course of reasoning to demonstrate the subordination of adaptation to individuation. He cites, as one example of frustrating adaptation, suicides like that of George Eastman, founder of Kodak, who took his life at the end of a successful career, leaving a note that read: "My work is done. Why wait?"

8 Another example is given in *L'open space m'a tuer*, by Alexandre des Isnards and Thomas Zuber (*op. cit.*): in some companies, employees are obliged to constantly change cubicles, to prevent them from acquiring a routine or friendships that might take up too much of their time. Again, the goal is never to allow the individual the luxury of being well-adapted. It seems that better results are obtained from workers who have to struggle to adapt.

endurance. Such limits certainly exist, and must be determined on a case-by-case basis. But more fundamentally, there is an ontological limit, which could be defined as the necessity of curbing adaptation in order to allow it to develop towards self-realization. It is the height of pointlessness to push towards endless adaptation without ever seeking self-realization, to concern ourselves only with the means, and never with the end.

Armed with this analysis, we can better appreciate the hypocrisy of so many managerial tracts that disguise their avaricious objectives with ennobling jargon, valorizing the practice of pushing people to their limits in order to extract the maximum profit from their efforts. These tracts have a common unifying theme: they transform environmental constraints into values. Instead of saying, "Adapt," they say, "Adopt new values." It sounds better that way. In a time when meaning is often situational, the language of values retains the comforting glow of authority. Thus, a woman trying to reconcile professional life and family life is transformed into an idealized icon, that of the "executive woman." Struggling to manage an excessive amount of work is labeled "positive stress," while consenting to be shuffled from one position to another is recast as "flexibility." Being presented with contradictory information is an opportunity to demonstrate "open-mindedness" and a capacity for "multi-dimensional thinking," while submitting to the quantification of employee performance is "evaluation."[9] Responding to endless emails full of requests and reminders is "being plugged-in," and keeping one's phone on at all times is "being reachable." Immediate compliance with all demands is called "responsiveness," while straining one's eyes for twelve hours a day in front of a computer screen is renamed "availability." In this way, a bizarre assortment of buzz-words keep us glued to our seats.

Everywhere, the language of values is flourishing. But the people who devise and employ it have misunderstood the concept: these

9 "Numbers don't have souls," writes Mathieu Terence. "They can easily be made to say things that words struggle to express without sounding false. Emanating from a different sphere than that of discourse, they are beyond reproach," in *Le Devenir du nombre*, Paris, Stock, 2012, p. 35.

propositions are not "values." Values are much less determinate and much more subject to interpretation than the Newspeak terminology embraced by corporate management teams. These would-be values are in fact thinly veiled orders, constraints by another name. The language of values pretends to operate on a different plain from the discourse of adaptation, but in reality, it is concerned with nothing else. The problem, again, is that the adaptations it engenders have no means of progressing toward self-realization. Locked into a cycle of repetition that ends in exhaustion, perfectionism finally runs out of steam: the work of perfecting an adaptation proves to be ultimately relentless and frustrating.

The worst adaptations are those that dominate in a world ruled by profits, where individuals are obliged to submit to diktats formulated far from their sphere of work, by people who are often oblivious to its rhythms and codes. More than ever before, a passion for money has overrun our planet, and its corollary—raw, materialistic egotism—is everywhere on display, unhindered by shame or restraint. Already, at the turn of the last century, Charles Péguy was decrying this trend, writing in his essay *On Money*:

> We are living with the most monstrous inequality ever seen in the history of the world. Or, we were living. We had children. They did not have the feeling that we have of being imprisoned. They did not have, as we do, the sense of economic strangulation, of an iron collar around our throats that tightens each day by one notch.[10]

His words still resonate today. Other figures have taken up the mantle from the powers he invokes; credit rating agencies, multinational companies and hedge funds have replaced the old constraints, but by no means has the iron collar stopped tightening, nor has the sense of strangulation subsided. On the contrary: as they become ever more "virtual" and "globalized," the pressure these powers exert becomes even crueler and more forceful. The key to the problem is their greed, which is the ultimate source of estrangement.

[10] Charles Péguy, *L'Argent* [*On Money*], reissued by Éditions des Équateurs, Paris, 2008.

Time is undoubtedly the most precious of our resources. "I seek the gold of time," wrote André Breton, who had this alchemical formula inscribed on his tombstone. Like him, many of us are eager to experience the most exciting things that time has to offer. But in the pathologies of civilization that we have been examining, time is transformed. The constraint of adaptation has taken over this dimension of our lives. The dominant theme of modern society is adaptation to temporal norms: to calendars, deadlines, timetables, meetings. Schedules are everywhere, time is nowhere. The term *deadline* reveals how morbid our concept of temporality has become. The deadline is the fatal, agonizing minute, the final moment after which all will be lost. Time has metamorphosed into a commodity whose depletion is a source of anxiety. It is strange to consider that our civilization has produced innumerable technological innovations intended to save us time, yet we so frequently find ourselves short on time that we are obliged to adopt a frenetic pace, just to maintain our existence. Acceleration has become a source of alienation, as has been observed by Hartmut Rosa, who, after Paul Virilio, is one of the first theorists to examine this cultural mutation. The "silent normative power of temporal norms"[11] forces us to adopt strategies that maximize speed, ultimately leaving us with the impression that we are not in control of our own lives. We seem to exist entirely within a framework of schedules that are externally imposed: train timetables, traffic patterns, work hours, school hours, lunch hours, childcare hours, store opening and closing times, television schedules, bedtimes and wake-up times; all of our time is locked into place.

And yet, luxuriating in time is one of our greatest occasions for intimacy with ourselves and with the world. We can experience a sense of communion with our environment only when we enter into a peaceable relationship with temporality, in which the passage of time is a gift to be shared, a source of symbiosis and an opportunity for

[11] Hartmut Rosa, *Aliénation et accélération. Vers une théorie critique de la modernité tardive*, Paris, La Découverte, 2012, p. 57. [Originally published in German as *Beschleunigung: Die Veränderung der Zeitstrukturen in der Moderne*, Frankfurt am Main Suhrkamp, 2005. Published in English as *Social Acceleration: A New Theory of Modernity*, trans. Jonathan Trejo-Mathys, New York, Columbia University Press, 2013.]

observation. Through this passage of time, this duration, as Bergson calls it, life becomes a perpetual state of creation. It is no longer a matter of adapting ourselves to time, but of using our time to construct an interior life that is rich, surprising, and even visionary. Time is not our enemy. It is the very fabric of our lives. It turns hostile only when, segmented and compartmentalized, it becomes a vector through which lives are controlled and exploited. It is this phenomenon that gives rise to what Hartmut Rosa describes as "pathologies of desynchronization," about which he writes:

> Authors like Alain Ehrenberg and Lothar Baier have explained the spectacular increase in the number of cases of depression and burnout as an apparent reaction to the increased time pressures and elevated stress levels of modern society. In fact, as people enter into a state of depression, they experience a sudden change in their perception of time; what had seemed fluid and dynamic now feels viscous and stagnant. They are plunged into a temporal quagmire, where time no longer seems to move forward. Any meaningful connection between past, present and future is completely destroyed.[12]

"Work without end" is an expression with a double meaning: it may indicate the absence of a limit or the absence of finality. In practice, these two deregulations often go together, culminating in a loss of momentum. Nor do they only concern the sphere of work. The absence of limits and of finality more generally characterizes the darker side of our technological civilization. Here again, burnout is the reflection of the society that causes it. Overload is also a defining factor in the consumption of technology and other commodities. In a world where consumers are expected to spend money they don't have on products they don't need to impress people they don't like, overindulgence is everywhere; meaning is nowhere. Overwork for some results from a frenzy of consumption on the part of others, provoked by the voracious financial appetites of a third group. The entire system is defined by *excess*. The cycles of frenzied activity and subsequent depletion are a

[12] *Ibid.*, p. 95.

global phenomenon, and the mechanisms for abuse of adaptation also operate on a global scale.

What is technology, after all, if not a tool for adapting to the world? Technologies are a means. They were developed to serve human beings, not to enslave them. Yet the proliferation of technologies, which are, individually, amazing cultural achievements, has led to the creation of a complex "technical environment" to which each of us must adapt. This environment has its own laws and its own requirements. It is evolving rapidly. For those who are able to adapt, it can be generous on a material level, providing comfort and security. But adaptation comes at a high price. Conforming to the demands of this technical environment has a financial cost, which the individual must work hard to afford. Since the technical environment is constantly increasing in complexity, it must be met with ever more time-consuming and costly strategies. These strategies are not insurmountable, in and of themselves. Indeed, enthusiastic technophiles can boast of a technical environment made by people, for people, which is, in essence, the realization of our fantasies, at once the beginning and the end of our illusions. All we have to do is adapt, stay up to date, evolve with the times. To what end, we might ask? In order to be well-adapted, of course. And why? In order to stay inside the system, to reap its latest benefits and, above all, to be ready for the next set of updates. Here again, the tyranny of adaptation has no end beyond its own perpetuation. The means form a barrier that blocks out any glimpse of a final goal.

Here too, there is an urgent need for a pact with technology. These problems, which are in all respects philosophical, reveal the inescapable influence of a technologized society and its norms. What, after all, is the model for a set of behaviors that are perfectly adapted, but in no way concerned with self-realization? The only convincing answer is: the operation of a technical object. When we expect workers to manifest unquestioning perfectionism, our unconscious motivation is often the desire to make people resemble machines—reliable, polyvalent, and soulless. A new *mimesis* guides our business models. Since the technical object is an example of success, it serves more and more as a standard of comparison that we are expected to strive towards. In many professional contexts, it is a great compliment to say that someone works "like a machine."[13]

But this desire for resemblance cuts us off from our higher aspirations, confining us to the realm of functionality. If our reflections on burnout have led us to call for a pact with technology, one motivating factor is the need to dismantle this pattern of *mimesis*. Humans have created excellent machines. Our purpose in so doing was to benefit from them, not to resemble them; to work with them, not to emulate their performance. Our pact with technology must bear in mind this fundamental difference, which, in principle, no one would dare to publicly deny, but which, in practice, is often violated: human beings are creatures of desire, but also creatures of imperfection; we are inherently unspecialized. The hand, which Aristotle called "the tool of tools," lends itself to an endless variety of tasks. But, unlike the highly specialized organs of other animals, there is no gesture that it can execute with the monotonous consistency and absence of variation that are the hallmarks of perfection. The hand is the symbol of a creature that thrive's on variation and change, with an affinity for novelty that is facilitated by its lack of specialization. Any desire to resemble a machine or to make workers resemble them, is thus hopelessly regressive. In contrast, a pact with technology would allow us, as human beings, to appreciate this difference and to reaffirm our perfect imperfection.

Otherwise, we will be hearing the phrase "loss of meaning" more and more frequently. The expression is often used in cases of burnout, but it also crops up to describe the situation of consumers overwhelmed by an abundance of products, viewers reduced to a television-induced stupor, and lost souls wandering through the vast warehouses that used to be recognizable as shopping centers. For the philosopher, meaning is always difficult to define. It is everywhere, yet it resists isolation. Anyone who tries to grasp it winds up like the subway workers in Fellini's *Roma*.

13 Numerous echoes of this fantasy of mimesis can be found in the novel *Aprender a Rezar na Era da Técnica* [*Learning to Pray in the Age of Technique*], by the Portuguese novelist and epistemologist Gonçalo M. Tavares (published in French as *Apprendre à prier à l'ère de la technique*. Paris, Viviane Hamy, 2010).

Drilling a subterranean tunnel, they break through to an ancient Roman room whose magnificent frescos are momentarily illuminated by their flashlights. For one moment of grace, they contemplate these half-glimpsed marvels, before exposure to air causes them to oxidize, crack, and crumble to dust. Meaning is like those frescos. Its loss haunts us, but in its absence we can no longer explain it. It has an ineffable quality that changes everything but cannot be put into words. It is thus nearly impossible to speak directly about meaning, or the loss thereof. The topic must be approached in a roundabout way. We might ask ourselves, in the case at hand, whether meaning could be a certain equilibrium between the life-phases of adaptation and self-realization. If, in other words, meaning might be found in a successful oscillation between efforts to adapt to an environment and the contemplation of a world in which our work has been a source of satisfaction and serenity.

Adaptation for its own sake is pointless and absurd. Adaptation that culminates in self-realization has a meaning—one that we must pursue. How we conceive of adaptation in a complex world is exactly the issue that a pact with technology needs to address. A proposal for such a pact is broadly outlined at the conclusion of this book and developed in more detail in *L'âge des transitions.*[14] What is needed is a solution to the modern paradox that currently confounds us: the more technology there is, the more we humans have to adapt to it; but the more we adapt, the less freedom we have (and consequently, the more our new technologies can impose upon us). If transition presents us with a new way of framing this problem, it does so by letting us choose to see the means and the ends as equally important. In our goal-oriented society, we are often willing to embrace any technological means that moves us toward our ends. For example, it seems to matter little to us whether our energy source is petrol, the procurement of which may possibly have sparked a military conflict, or clean, renewable energy, as long as our cars keep moving forward. If we decide, instead, to scrupulously select the means we use based on ethics—whether environmentalist or

[14] P. Chabot, *L'âge des transitions* [*The Age of Transitions*], Paris, PUF, 2015.

convivialist in nature—the sense of being forced to adapt to a set of means imposed upon us is attenuated. In a technological civilization, the ends are, in fact, created by the means, which are, in the final analysis, the stuff from which our world is constructed. The idea of a pact with technology allows us to reconsider the means, restoring their importance and value (rather than letting them go all but unnoticed, as is typically the case in our consumption, which is concerned only with the satisfaction of our desires, by any means necessary), but also selecting means that are adapted to our human needs. And not the other way around . . .

The useful and the subtle

In a novel appropriately titled *Burn-out*, Patricia Martel describes the exhausting years she spent as a young intern at public hospitals, racking up night shifts and disillusionments. Her hopes were high, to begin with. But reality is sometimes more persistent than hope. One morning, between patient visits, a drug company sales rep arrived to extol the merits of a new antidepressant, Survivor 3®, with particular emphasis on the test that allowed the drug's inventors to induce a state of depression in rodents. A crucial breakthrough, he explained, was the "forced swimming test." Previous studies had employed the method known as "suspension by the tail," but it had to be conceded that this technique was considerably less effective than forced swimming at inducing a depressive state:

> It was observed that having to struggle against whatever was holding its tail tended, paradoxically, to make the animal more vigorous. In contrast, in the forced swimming test, there was no designated enemy! The animal was obliged to fight against itself. And experience shows that this method results in many more animals becoming rapidly discouraged.[15]

[15] Patricia Martel, *Burn-out*, Biarritz, Atlantica, 2010, p. 80.

No designated enemy! Just the need to keep swimming. Sink or swim. No one to blame, no metaphysical bureau of complaints. The book's heroine, who sees a parallel between the rats in the forced swimming test and her own struggle to stay afloat amidst the moans of ailing patients and the urgent questions of the dying, knows that the test is pitiless. Subjected to constant stress, isolation, and fear of failure, the young intern must stay strong for everyone. She even ends up having to console the sales rep, who explodes one day, and, at the climax of a spectacular nervous breakdown, turns against the very drug company executives whose coffers he has been lining:

> You know, eventually, they'll end up convincing us we're all bonkers! They'll make us believe that we all need drugs to stay sane, when it's the world that's gone crazy! Survivor, Survivor, yes, of course! They picked the right name! And what about real life, then? Where has it gone? Like my wife, it's there, and then it slips away from you.[16]

Everyone in this book, which is a work of fiction in name only, is suffering. The patients, first of all, but also the doctors and nurses, who all seem desperately in need of a week's relaxation on a sunny beach—or at least some additional support. One cannot help but think of Freudenberger, who came to the ego-bruising realization that in his own hospital, he was quite possibly more exhausted than any of his patients—the burnt-out case *par excellence*, surrounded by drug addicts who could at least find a bit of serenity between hits.

From the beginning, burnout has been disproportionately prevalent among members of the caring professions: medical personnel, as well as teachers and other educators. The first recorded cases affected these sectors.[17] It was only later that business professionals, both white collar and blue collar, came to join their ranks.

[16] *Ibid.*, p. 178.

[17] Recent statistics confirm that the caring professions still account for a significant percentage of all cases of burnout. See, for example, Suzanne Peters and Patrick Meesters, *Vaincre l'épuisement professionnel* [*Overcoming Professional Exhaustion*], Paris, Robert Laffont, 2007, p. 141.

Cynicism is a common manifestation of exhaustion. Each profession has its own particular means of expressing it. The doctor looks at her patient and says: "One way or another, you're going to wind up dead." The teacher calls his students idiots and gives up trying to teach them anything. As for the philosopher, her burnout is signaled by a discouraged attitude toward language. "These are only words; they won't change anything," she sighs, closing her book.[18] Freudenberger, for his part, cites the case of a teacher who alternated between tranquilizers and cannabis, to keep himself from insulting his own students. He also describes a nurse fed up with watching her patients die, and a social worker at a detox clinic who directs alcoholics to the nearest bar. The cynicism barely obscures their underlying anger and frustration. The Shakespearean adage about hoisting oneself with one's own petard comes to mind. How better to convey that the first victims of cynicism are the cynics themselves, who destroy whatever is most precious to them in order to express their own sense of powerlessness?

Why does burnout affect the caring professions disproportionately? We might actually have expected them to be spared from this affliction, since professional exhaustion has been purported to coincide with a loss of meaning, like the acedic's loss of faith, and it is hard to imagine a profession with a more self-evident signification than teaching or medicine. The notion that such a loss could manifest itself on a school playground, at the bedside of an ailing patient, or even in a maternity ward, disconcerts us. If the thing that gives work meaning is a sense of connection to other people, working in one of these places should be inherently meaningful. Yet it is in precisely such situations that meaninglessness is most keenly felt. This is where the problem first surfaces. But, why?

The most basic explanation is that to care for people is to watch them suffer, and to come face to face with fragility and imperfection. Illness is always a source of stress. A child's failure to thrive academically can have weighty consequences. The psychiatrist Alexis Burger has noted

[18] One might reread Wittgenstein's *Tractatus* in light of this observation.

that it is often necessary to override one's natural instincts in order to remain in a caregiver role with someone who is suffering:

> In a stress-inducing situation, the natural behavior exhibited by animals is a fight or flight response. But, in a care-based relationship, which, by definition, represents a concentration of difficult interactions, one can neither escape nor attack; one is obligated to stay, even if one finds it unbearable.[19]

Those who seek to help others are caught up in three simultaneous struggles. They struggle with the problems of those they are trying to care for or educate. They wrestle with elements of their own personalities, including sensitivity, countertransference, and discouragement. And finally, they must face the pressures of a society in which mercy and compassion are seldom seen as high priorities.

To bolster these observations, we may recall Freud's famous remark that there are three impossible professions: teaching, healing, and governing. Eighty years later, the first two of these professions account for the largest number of burnout cases. The father of psychoanalysis first expressed this idea in 1925, repeating it in 1937 in *Analysis Terminable and Interminable*, with the comment that these are vocations "in which one can be sure beforehand of achieving unsatisfying results."[20] Freud did not invent the notion of impossible professions. It came from a popular German saying that made humorous reference to this impossibility. The three professions in question all revolve around human relationships, by means of which they seek to modify the behavior of others. These are vocations inherently linked to people, in contrast to technical or material pursuits. Educational, therapeutic and

[19] Alexis Burger, "Comment devenir un meilleur professionnel en se protégeant [How to become a Better Professional by Protecting Yourself]," in *Repère social*, no 19, July 2000, cited by Catherine Vasey in *Burn-out: le détecter et le prévenir* [*Detecting and Preventing Burnout*], Geneva, Jouvence, 2009.

[20] Sigmund Freud, "Analysis Terminable and Interminable," in *International Journal of Psycho-Analysis*, Vol. 18, Psychoanalytic Electronic Publishing, 2012, p. 401. For a reflection on this theme, see M. Fain, J. Cournut, E. Enriquez and M. Cifali, *Les Trois Métiers Impossibles* [*The Three Impossible Professions*], Paris, Les Belles Lettres, 1987, as well as the work of August Aichhorn.

political relationships all have the objective of changing other people, who may well resist modification and whose resistance may even be essential to their construction of an autonomous identity. Acting for the good of others may turn out be "the worst tyranny imaginable," as Kant put it. It's not hard to understand why Freud found success under these circumstances to be inevitably "unsatisfying." In moments of doubt, the teacher, the doctor, and the politician all run up against the fatal question, to which there may be no answer: "What right do I have to impose my own truth upon others?"

And yet, these three vocations were the bulwarks of classical humanism. They epitomize the ideals that Plato and Aristotle envisioned for a virtuous and healthy citizen in a just city-state. The very professions that Freud identified as impossible, and from which Freudenberger drew his first patients, had, for twenty centuries, been central to European culture and its concern for human dignity. In this context, burnout can again be seen to reflect the dysfunctionalities of the era in which it appears. It is a symptom of the difficulty of caring for, educating, and civilizing individuals in a technology-driven society. This modern problem afflicts that which is most precious to us.

Burnout is a testament to the exhaustion of humanism. It is the sign of the deep conflict that has emerged in our time between two forms of progress. For, if the postmodern world continues to be shaped by the ideology of development, it also remains divided as to the nature of this development. It tries, with limited success, to reconcile two different types of "advancement": useful progress and subtle progress. A powerful image that illustrates the tension between these two types of progress emerges in Maylis de Kerangal's novel *Birth of a Bridge*. Her book, set in an unnamed Latin-American country, describes how the banks of an immense river are transformed by the vision of the mayor of the town of Coca, who is determined, after a visit to Dubai, "to be finished with the slow, the old, the broken down."[21] He decides to commission the

[21] Maylis de Kerangal, *Birth of a Bridge* (*La naissance d'un pont*), trans. Jessica Moore, Vancouver, Talonbooks, 2014, p. 43.

construction of a giant bridge, nineteen hundred meters in length, which will run between two enormous towers and will make use of two million tons of concrete, eighty thousand tons of steel, and one hundred and twenty-nine thousand kilometers of cables.

> Bringing these two landscapes together—there, that's the site, that's the story: electric sintering, reconciliation, fluidizing of powers, elaboration of a relationship, this is what there is to do, this is the job . . .[22]

Kerangal's novel is an ode to the useful, recounting the saga of the bridge workers who arrive from all directions to dredge the river, operate cranes, mix concrete and, finally, to provide a full-scale validation of the thousands of hours spent by its designers in planning its every detail. This metaphor for the labor of modern humanity depicts it as an epic endeavor, launching an enormous bridge towards the future.

Alongside this *useful* undertaking, Kerangal's novel also brings to life the stories of individual people. Minute and inconsequential in comparison with the edifice of concrete and steel that towers above them, they are nonetheless its *raison d'être*: the people who will make use of it—engineers, construction workers and their families, the native population who view it with suspicion, and the mayor who seeks to profit from it. Within this ordinary human comedy, the same eternal motifs are played out: love, hate, childhood, jealousy . . . They appear all too familiar against the backdrop of the enormous bridge, with its pure lines and clear guiding principles. But they represent humanity, in all of its warmth and imprecision. It, too, is progressing, but to the rhythm of a different, subtler logic.

Embodied by the bridge, the type of useful progress that holds sway in the sciences, in technology, and in material culture, is driven by the accumulation of capital. In this sphere, each new insight, invention, or discovery propels further innovation. Each artefact contributes to an ever-increasing store of capital that humankind draws upon to improve its knowledge base and overall well-being. The exponential and multilinear trajectory of technological progress can be explained by the

[22] *Ibid.*, p. 63.

snowball effect: computers keep getting smaller and more complex because each new generation of electronic devices inherits positive characteristics from the previous generation. To be sure, in this multilinear process, some things are lost or forgotten. But they are incidental to the ultimate goal of this enterprise: to make existence profitable.

Occurring alongside this useful progress is a type of "subtle" development whose laws are shaped by the spirit of finesse, rather than geometry, and whose sphere of application is humanity, rather than the material world. Progress is not, in fact, confined to the realm of science and technology. It was a strategic error on the part of the humanists not to contest the notion that the material world alone could be the source of advancement. Certain intellectuals have since seen fit to denounce our progress-oriented civilization, adopting the world-weary posture of those who have given up on the illusion of development. But in so doing, they have ceded the course to the proponents of useful progress, who have been left alone to propel humanity toward a better future, and to determine what this "better" future should look like. A different approach is needed, one that does not consist of opposing useful progress with a kind of nihilistic irenicism, or of ridiculing even the most desperate attempts to improve the lot of humankind. For if not that, then what? A return to the age of hunter-gatherers is not a viable option. It would be more fruitful to restore and nurture, along with useful progress, a "subtle progress" that centers around individuals, their education, their way of living and caring for themselves, the treatment of their neuroses, and the prioritization of their happiness. These endeavors also engender a kind of progress, albeit less tangible than its useful counterpart.

This subtle progress does not benefit from the robustness of a system based on exponentially increasing capital. It is driven not by the snowball effect, but by a process of initiation, which must start anew each time it is implemented. This type of progress is the realm of new beginnings, like in Kerangal's novel, where each individual character has to learn how to live. Knowledge, where human matters are concerned, is always acquired gradually, because it is nothing without experience. In the subtlest areas of human progress—specifically, in the quest to achieve a balance between passion and tranquility in our relationship with the world—advancement is impossible without the investment of time. Education is the fruit of patience. It is the opposite of instant gratification. To use a contemporary example that encapsulates the tension between these two concurrent systems, it is impossible to download the contents of a teacher's brain into the mind of a student. The solution is not a technological one. More to the point, there is no "solution," because there is no "problem." There is only life, which continues from one generation to the next, and which is the foundation for all forms of humanism.[23]

This is where burnout comes in, as a symptom of the conflict between the two types of progress. The fragile human sphere faces enormous pressure from technological and economic forces. The results it produces will never be as manifest as a superb bridge or a productive factory. It is not profitable; it cannot be expected to yield enormous dividends. On the contrary, subtle progress always skirts the edge of the abyss. It operates within a realm of extremes, of beginnings and endings. A young mother leans toward her child as it babbles its first words. A teacher transmits knowledge to students distracted by their own vain efforts to find themselves within the immensity of the world's memory. A doctor attempts to explain to her patient that everything is finite, paraphrasing the illness itself, verbalizing the cyclical nature of life. What these professions have in common is that they help us to live. They accompany us in our subtle progress along the path of existence, never shying away from the tragic aspects of the human condition: ignorance, death, loss, stupidity.

But, in a society that ecstatically greets the triumph of useful progress, this confrontation with the fragility of beginnings appears anachronistic. Useful progress knows nothing of the abyss. It is oblivious to cycles and unconcerned with the delicate problems of origins. It flourishes in a state of exponential development, a fact which is not without consequence for

[23] For further discussion of the links between the useful and the subtle, see P. Chabot, *Les Sept Stades de la philosophie* [*The Seven Stages of Philosophy*], Paris, PUF, 2011.

its adherents, who, to put it bluntly, sometimes grow impatient with humanity. This ideology is in evidence on the websites of the modern-day millenarians known as transhumanists:[24] having to die, to undertake the risky process of reproduction, to produce successive generations who will in turn be obliged to relearn the rules of grammar and spelling—the atavism and imprecision of these activities is typical of an aging species in need of an upgrade. If the transhumanists want to improve our species, it is because they are disheartened by its present condition. Accustomed to computers and stringent technical standards, they see our attempts at living as clumsy and amateurish. All of this must change, they think to themselves. It fuels their fantasies. Observing the young, nearly burnt-out instructor tasked with teaching grammar to a class full of teenagers who would rather be left to their own devices, they assure themselves that one day we will be able to format young brains with the relevant syntactical rules, just as we do computers … And similarly, confronted with dying patients who wearily close their eyes in the fading light, transhumanists tell themselves that it is time to interrupt these perpetual beginnings and endings, this peregrination of living beings who blossom and then perish. Their dreams are not unlike those of the monks of an earlier age, who imagined a world beyond to mitigate the vicissitudes of the world they knew. Their fantasies conform to principles that have become the slogans of our times: expand the empire of the techno-sciences and apply the rationality that guides it to its human approximation.[25]

24 "Transhumanism" refers here to the intellectual movement which maintains that our human limitations can and should be overcome only by means of techno-scientific interventions (prostheses, implants, gene therapy, psychoactive substances, etc.). For a more detailed account of the differences between transhumanism, post-humanism and other expressions of the desire to "go beyond" humanity, a yearning already articulated, in different ways, by both Nietzsche and Foucault, see G. Hottois and J.N. Missa, *L'humain et ses préfixes*, Paris, Vrin, 2016.

25 Nikolaus Geyrhalter's documentary *Donauspital* (2012), illustrates this metaphysical impatience with human limitations. In filming one of Europe's biggest hospitals, the *Donauspital* in Vienna, he unveils a futuristic ballet featuring robots, high-tech scanners, and semi-automated operating rooms. The irony exposed by his camera is the contrast between the precision and efficiency of the technology and the fragility of the ailing, bed-ridden, human patients. The imbalance between the useful and the subtle is reinforced by his decision not to record any dialogue. Nevertheless, we can imagine that as soon as speech resumes, the balance of power will shift, and the domain of the subtle will again give rise to invention.

But members of the caring professions are not fooled. They know that they have devoted themselves to the most difficult domain. They are not oblivious to the fact that the realm of beginnings and endings, and indeed, the cyclical nature of life itself, is a reality that contemporary society keeps repressed. They feel the moral pressure that this repression imposes on them as the last defenders of an increasingly problematic form of humanism. Our society's philosophical impatience with the human condition is palpable, and we are quick to remind carers that their contribution to real human advancement is relatively minor—for example, by offering them salaries that just barely allow them to pay the bills. Money stays in the domain of useful progress: financial capital and technological capital reinforce one another. Instrumental logic further imposes on the caring professions the burden of supplementary administrative tasks and the need to justify their performance in financial terms. The domain of the subtle has been colonized. Those who are left to defend its borders are showing signs of strain.

Here again, we must conceive of a pact with technology as a means for modern-day humans to re-establish a balance between useful and subtle progress. For if the latter is fragile, the former, by itself, is all but meaningless. The exhaustion of humanism, of which burnout is a symptom, ultimately stems from an imbalance between these two forms of evolution. If this inequality persists and deepens, technological and economic interests will eventually subsume the interests of the human beings who gave rise to them. This is why a new pact is necessary, to protect humanity from its own capacity for self-destruction, just as in the eighteenth century, the idea of a social contract served to defend society from endogenous risks of implosion.

Only a pact of this nature would allow us to bring an end to the epidemic of discouragement that has been ravaging the caring professions. If Freud was right to say that teaching, healing, and governing are "impossible" pursuits, it must be added that these very impossibilities are the basis of our freedom and our dignity as human beings. Instead of trying to do without them, we would do better to look to them as a source of creativity and pleasure, for within them is all that is most precious to us. Humankind must be protected from itself, in order to preserve the delicate balance that we, at our best, are capable of maintaining between the fragile and the powerful, the subtle and the useful.

Recognition and disregard

What do business executives at multinational companies think about during their daily meetings? Ongoing projects, stocks and dividends, organizational restructuring, layoffs, and a thousand other details, as well: a neighbor's tie, the boss's worried expression, the nervous gestures of a co-worker. And then, beyond the strictly professional sphere, the minds of the participants wander, when they can, onto more private subjects: problems at home, travel plans, fantasies. Meetings constitute peculiar moments in time. The activities of each individual in attendance come to a halt for the sake of a cooperative endeavor that is by no means free from judgement, mind games, settling of scores, or ambition-fueled power struggles. Some participants can be seen exchanging nudges, while others hope they won't be asked to speak. Everyone puts his or her best foot forward. But behind their placid faces, in the deepest reaches of their minds, discordant voices are murmuring.

In *Marge brute* [*Gross Margin*], Laurent Quintreau employs the most intimate and intrusive of literary techniques to capture the thoughts of eleven executives trapped in a management meeting. By means of interior monologues, he gives us access to the private, uncensored discourse that each of them is conducting in his or her head. Inside the secret citadels of these corporate minds, things are, as depicted by Quintreau, uglier and less controlled than we might have been led to believe. Some are libidinous, others cynical. One is holding back tears, another is shivering and nauseous. All of them are secretly at war with one another. Their suppressed frustrations give rise to harsh judgements that their coded conversations only hint at. These representatives of the working world are base, power-hungry, and vulgar. They are supposedly working on cutting-edge developments. But as specimens of humanity, they are decidedly under-developed.

This is an unsettling book. The reality is no doubt different—better, or worse. Nonetheless, in capturing the interior monologues of these characters, Quintreau has brought into the open all of the unspoken words, unrealized desires, irrational cruelties, ambitions, fears, and lies that motivate a group of people gathered around the same table, not for reasons of mutual appreciation, but because they happen to work together. Every facet of human nature is to be found there. But, if the literature on the topic is to be believed, what we will find there most of all is a common desire, deeply felt, though differently expressed in the mind of each: the desire for recognition.

The hunger for recognition seems to be one of the most universal of all modern-day preoccupations. We hear it articulated by a plugged-in, young executive: "I'm not even forty, I'm the youngest one here, I process situations at lightning speed, I'm an exceptional guy . . ."; by an HR director nearing the end of her career: "soon I'll be tossed out like an old rag—me, the hard-working, model employee, who always gave everything she had for this business, who was never stingy with her time or her energy when the company's interests were on the line . . ."; by a working mother trying to convince herself that she has everything under control: " I'm not anxious, not anymore; my portfolios are up to date, and my beneficiary accounts; my heart is beating normally; those tranquilizers were really effective . . ."; or by an intern wondering if he's chosen the wrong profession: "I don't want to end up bitter like them; this is the second place I've worked, and it's always the same, misery and resentment from top to bottom. There's still time to turn back, shift gears, change course, ok, but where else can I go . . ."[26] All of them are devising strategies that are sure to get them recognized. After salary, recognition is the most coveted form of compensation in the working world.

In cases of burnout, complaints about denial of recognition are common. But what is meant by this notion? What lies behind it? What

[26] Laurent Quintreau, *Marge brute*, Paris, Denoël, 2006, pp. 65, 98, 15 and 107.

are we really looking for, when we chase after recognition? Recognition is the symbolic counterpart to the work we perform. It is, first of all, an acknowledgement, notes Christophe Dejours,[27] a confirmation that its recipient is a valuable contributor to a professional organization, and that, without his or her participation, certain tasks would remain undone. It is, furthermore, an expression of gratitude for services rendered, a sort of all-purpose "thank you" that isn't tied to a particular accomplishment, but simply acknowledges the fact that a particular person spends some significant portion of his or her life working for other people. Upon examination, being compelled, day in and day out, to dedicate the better part of one's energies to a business or an institution is no trivial matter. Philosophically, this constitutes a gift of the self, a sacrifice of one's time, which is truly the most precious thing an individual has to offer. When the hours run out, we will have nothing left. By giving our time to someone else, we deplete our most intimate store of capital, without which everything else we own is worthless. From this perspective, it makes sense that recognition understood as gratitude would be so fervently sought after. Only a symbolic compensation could be metaphysically commensurate with this gift of the self. Only a sincere "thank you" could effectively acknowledge the unnaturalness of giving such a significant portion of one's days to someone else.[28] Human beings who must, by necessity, do violence to their own sense of self, want to see this sacrifice highlighted. They want to know that their offering has not gone unnoticed. This is the source of that immense hunger for recognition which, when unfulfilled, provokes a visceral feeling of resentment. It is a typical underlying cause of professional exhaustion.

[27] Christophe Dejours, *Travail vivant 2*, *op. cit.*, p. 104.

[28] For an analysis of the theme of recognition as reciprocation for a gift-offering, see Alain Caillé, "Sur la reconnaissance [On Recognition]," in A. Caillé (ed.), *La Quête de reconnaissance. Nouveau phénomène social total* [*The Quest for Recognition: a Completely New Social Phenomenon*], Paris, La Découverte, 2007: "The theory of the individual in search of recognition is likely to prove identical to that of the giver, the individual who enters the cycle of giving, receiving and giving back again. A sociological theory of recognition would have to be anti-utilitarian, or else it wouldn't be."

Practically speaking, recognition only occasionally takes on these metaphysical dimensions. It is more often manifested in the form of judgements, which assess both the utility of the work performed and the beauty of the resulting product. In this way, it remains anchored in reality, focusing first on the concrete results of the work completed, then shifting focus toward the person who completed it. Thus, the chef is complimented on the flavor of the food she prepares, the electrician for his expert placement of overlapping wires, the orator for the quality of her speeches. Such expressions of appreciation are even more valuable when proffered by one's peers, who are attuned to the arcane minutia of the task at hand, and thus most aware of the particular challenges it poses. For a layperson, putting a band-aid on a wound is an inconsequential act. For a nurse, it is a gesture which, when clumsily executed, can cause a patient unnecessary pain. Recognition expressed as a judgment of beauty is really a way of acknowledging a "fine piece of work," a notion originally applied to artisanal products, but which continues to be used today to describe even the most advanced technologies. Thus, there are, in computer science, "beautiful" lines of code, and in aeronautics, "perfect forms."

Hannah Arendt, who made a hierarchical and dichotomous distinction between "work" and "labor," erred in allowing class prejudice to influence her philosophy. For her, labor is repetitive, meaningless, purely functional. Work, in contrast, provides a platform for individual expression, an opportunity for the realization of a creative destiny. Starting from such propositions, one can understand why she would undervalue labor, especially physical labor, while elevating work, especially in the form of artistic or literary expression. But the fundamental premises of her argument are false, the ideological products of an excessively intellectual, and thus myopic worldview. The capacity to produce beautiful work is not restricted to any particular domain. Some gardeners display infinitely more artistry in their pruning of bushes than do certain hack writers in spewing out their novels. The distinction between work and labor is non-existent. The quality of work produced is a function of what the worker invests in it.

Christophe Dejours has a powerful way of conceptualizing the impact of recognition. He describes it as a means by which suffering can be transformed into pleasure.[29] Effort, exertion, and fatigue are unavoidable aspects of professional life, but they cannot be all there is to it. They must undergo a transformation. Recognition gives meaning to the hardships endured, confirming that the effort was not in vain, that it has led to a positive outcome. Unlike masochism, which eroticizes pain itself, this is not a case of suffering savored for its own sake. Instead, it is the recognition of suffering that transmutes it into its opposite, pleasure. This is a formidable act, one that can, in fact, be linked to a formulation of meaning. When the final result meets with approval, all the tensions and setbacks that preceded become meaningful: they were the obstacles that had to be overcome to produce a greater sense of satisfaction. Victory without peril brings triumph, but no glory. Dejours, being a psychoanalyst, goes so far as to connect this notion to the Freudian concept of sublimation, since in both cases, a compulsion is successfully channeled towards an activity that meets with society's approval.

In cases of burnout where lack of recognition is a primary contributing factor, this transformation of suffering into pleasure ceases to occur.[30] The sufferer can no longer transcend her fatigue, or view it positively. Its meaning escapes her, leaving her exhausted twice over: from working, first of all, but also from working in vain. This situation can arise from an assortment of causes, which may, in some cases, be intra-psychic. People who are habitually hard on themselves, reluctant to acknowledge any source of enjoyment, may find it impossible to leave the sphere of suffering for that of pleasure. Work is a source of

29 Christophe Dejours, *Travail vivant 2, op. cit.*, p. 107.

30 Dejours: "A lack of recognition is demotivating, and can give rise to a range of pathological conditions, including depression, mental confusion, paranoia, and self-harm" ("Psychanalyse et psychodynamique du travail: ambiguïtés de la reconnaissance [Psychoanalysis and Psychodynamics of Work: Ambiguities of Recognition]"), in Alain Caillé (ed.), *La Quête de reconnaissance* [*The Quest for Recognition*], *op. cit.*, p. 64. For more on this topic, see also Marie Pezé's impressive "consultation journal," *Ils ne mouraient pas tous mais tous étaient frappés* [*They didn't all die, but all were stricken*] (Paris, Flammarion, 2010), as well as Pascale Molinier's book, *Les enjeux psychiques du travail* [*The Psychological Stakes of Work*], Paris, Payot, 2006, particularly with regard to invisible activities such as domestic labor, which go unrecognized because they remain unseen (p. 145).

pain to them, and however much its positive aspects are emphasized, they will still approach it as a trial to be endured.

Lack of recognition can also be attributed—and this accounts for the majority of cases—to hierarchical organizations that disregard the need for it. Requests for recognition are sometimes brushed aside by those who see the desire for external validation as pointless and pathetic. Yet, in their refusal to recognize the efforts of others, they negate one of the essential elements of activity—the principle of cooperation—clinging instead to the hierarchical framework that protects them. Some of them, moreover, are so self-obsessed that they only see in others that which can serve their interests.

The dynamics of recognition can also be deliberately dismantled by hierarchical organizations that do not wish, either for strategic reasons or out of sheer perversity, to gratify their personnel with so much as a word of encouragement or praise. There may be advantages to leaving expectations of reward ungratified. Benjamin Constant makes an observation to this effect in a diary entry from 1804:

> In general, I have observed that it is advisable to thank people as infrequently as possible, because showing them recognition readily persuades them that they are doing too much! More than once, I have seen people stop themselves in the middle of performing a good deed, because, in their excessive gratitude, the recipients of their kindness made it out to be more than it was.[31]

As for the intentional, systematic withholding of recognition, it is one of the most violently irresponsible abuses of power. Recognition is central to the construction of a person's identity. Individual development within a society, or in the microcosm of the office, hinges upon the way in which a person is perceived. To deprive people of all consideration, oscillating instead between denigration, contempt, and disregard, is to attack the core of their being and strip them of self-confidence. These circumstances can set off some of the most severe pathological

[31] Benjamin Constant, *Journal intime.*

disorders. Yet, such strategies of intentional disregard are part of the protocol for certain businesses. The practice of "breaking" people is not the result of individual caprice. It is representative of a style of management which employs terror as a cost-cutting strategy, to precipitate the departure of employees who are already slated to be let go. The suicide epidemics that have occurred at certain companies reveal the full extent of the horror. It is imperative that regulations be put in place to penalize companies whose management techniques make strategic use of intimidation and psychological harassment.[32] Recent rulings by the French judicial system seem to be heading in this direction.

Nonetheless, the concept of recognition has been subject to criticism from a number of sources. The criticisms fall into two general categories. The first critique is Nietzschean, having been appropriated from that great German philosopher, or rather, a caricatured version of him, by certain business managers who extol the virtues of combat. In *Beyond Good and Evil*, Nietzsche criticizes the need for recognition as a notion typical of the morality of slaves, who await the judgement of others in order to know their own worth.[33] This objection, implicitly aimed at Hegel and his master–slave dialectic, is based on the conviction that a strong, aristocratic spirit need not submit to the opinion that others have of him. The master is the determiner of his own worth. The vulnerability and acceptance of suffering that lie behind a request for recognition are, in this view, characteristic of a weak-willed society overly concerned with social cohesion.

As for the second criticism, it has been put forward and subsequently neutralized by Axel Honneth, who has produced some of the most

32 See especially Jean-Philippe Desbordes' exploration of predatory management tactics in *Management circus. Une critique du management à l'époque postmoderne* [*Management Circus: A Critique of Management in the Postmodern Age*], Arles, Actes Sud, 2012. One interviewee confides: "I take responsibility for what I am and I don't feel any guilt about what I've accomplished. I've fulfilled my duties. I managed by terror, I picked out the weak links. It's true, there were some cases of suicide, but what could I do? The law today is survival of the fittest. Our whole world is deregulated now" (p. 15).

33 Friedrich Nietzsche, *Beyond Good and Evil*, London, Penguin Books, 1973, chapter 9, paragraph 261.

rigorous work on the topic of recognition. He has accurately observed that recognition, in the guise of flattery, can become an ideological weapon used to confine individuals to subservient positions and keep them from advancing. The purpose of the manoeuver is to build up a positive self-image among members of the targeted group, leading them to accept difficult tasks or put up with hardships. Hence, the praise received by soldiers who act courageously in battle increases in proportion to the perilousness of the next day's mission. Honneth gives another example:

> The appeals to the "good" mother and housewife made by churches, parliaments or the mass media over the centuries caused women to remain trapped within a self-image that most effectively accommodated the gender-specific division of labour.[34]

One can, likewise, massage employees' egos, assuring them that they are "independent workers," in order to demand from them more flexibility and tolerance for stress. Bolstered by this encouraging rhetoric, they do not dare to object or protest. In such situations, recognition is not liberating. It normalizes a difficult situation and makes it appear acceptable. Honneth's counter-argument begins by affirming that this type of ideological recognition amounts to an empty promise that is not supported by the attitudes of those who pay it lip service, let alone by financial compensation. When recognition is used solely for purposes of manipulation, the remuneration received is always purely rhetorical.

These criticisms must be taken into consideration, but they should not be seen to invalidate the concept of recognition, which is more relevant today than ever before. It is one of the essential elements of the new humanism which must serve as the antidote to our techno-capitalist age. As Hegel observed, recognition is a struggle. The combat has, in our time, taken various forms. Recognition has become the object of intense competition. And if the human need for recognition has grown so insistent, it is because people today are constantly confronted with

[34] Axel Honneth, "Recognition as Ideology," in A. Honneth, *The I in We: Studies in the Theory of Recognition*, Polity Press, Cambridge, 2012, p. 77.

powerful forces of depersonalization. Social networks, the perfect tools for manipulating appearances, are there to reassure and flatter us, providing us with thousands of friends and propping up our egos with positive affirmations . . . It's enough to almost give us the impression that we exist. And then, of course, there are the product brands, always there to remind us that everyone is different, that every act of consumption is an assertion of identity. In the words of Peter Sloterdijk:

> Which life should we try? Which flight should we book? We lose our footing because we have to choose from fourteen different types of salad dressing. The world is a menu: the point is to order and not to despair. That is the foundation of the postmodern condition.[35]

In this immense universe, each of us wants to be singled out and called by name. But the world is wide, and increasingly overpopulated, and we must often settle for being selected from an endless series of automated lists, into which our social security numbers and credit card information have already been entered. The watchwords of today's commercial propaganda are "respect and recognition." The "narcissism industry" that puts instant stardom within the reach of any internet user, thanks to the publicity provided by social media, is a good example of this: it assures all of us that we are "unique." Why, then, are so many of us still suffering? Why do we still feel cruelly ignored? Because that type of recognition is not the genuine article. We sense that it is superficial and calculating. Our desires as human beings are more profound. We want to be considered as individuals, not as consumers, nor as cogs in a machine that strips us of our individuality in order to make us conform to expectations. In a complex world where we often feel as anonymous as water droplets in a vast ocean, our quest for concrete signs of recognition is altogether understandable.

Recognition from an abstract entity doesn't satisfy our needs. What we need is a celebration of the ineffable qualities that make us human and give meaning to our pursuits.

35 Peter Sloterdijk, *Falls Europa erwacht* [*If Europe Awakes*], Frankfurt, Suhrkamp, 1994, p. 20; published in French as *Si l'Europe s'éveille*, Paris, Mille et Une Nuits, 1994, p. 32.

Women's burnout

Virginia Woolf maintained that every woman should have "a room of her own." In the main room of the house, with men casting inquisitive glances over her shoulder and children demanding constant attention, a woman was all too rarely granted the concentration necessary for creative work.

> Jane Austen . . . had no separate study to repair to, and most of the work must have been done in the general sitting-room, subject to all kinds of casual interruptions. She was careful that her occupation should not be suspected by servants or visitors or any persons beyond her own family party.[36]

A few square meters in which to work, free from male interference, might have made all the difference in the world. Yet, a century later, in open-plan offices, behind reception desks, at supermarket cash registers, or under the surveillance of video cameras that monitor assembly line production, many women must still dream of the private space that Virginia Woolf so ardently wished for them.[37]

Female workers, who still receive lower salaries than men performing the same tasks, are also more vulnerable than men to the scrutiny of the system. They are, furthermore, according to most studies, more often afflicted by burnout. Some years after coining the concept of professional exhaustion, Freudenberger co-wrote the book *Women's Burnout* with Gail North. Freudenberger and North recorded numerous first-hand accounts from women who reported sentiments like: "I had only one desire . . . I wanted to sit in a corner, put a paper bag over my head and

[36] Virginia Woolf, *A Room of One's Own*, New York, Harcourt, 2005, p. 66.

[37] "The transparency of spaces has various effects, writes Élisabeth Pélegrin-Genel: it makes production processes visible, maximizes productivity, prevents intimacies from forming, and reminds workers of their own transparency. In the working world, the stockholders are physically absent, the customers are at a distance, only the employees remain confined to their identical, duplicated spaces." For further discussion, see Pélegrin-Genel's excellent book *Des souris dans un labyrinthe. Décrypter les ruses et manipulations de nos espaces quotidiens* [*Rats in a Maze: Decrypting the Ruses and Manipulations of our Everyday Spaces*], Paris, La Découverte, 2010, p. 177.

say 'Leave me alone, world,' cause I'm not here.'"[38] Here again, a room of one's own becomes a longed-for refuge. But it is a refuge sought out of tearful desperation, and only an extended stay within its confines can restore the body to its habitual level of functionality. The presence of the external system isn't easy to forget. Like the eye of God in Victor Hugo's poem "La conscience," which haunts Cain as he tries in vain to flee from his own guilty conscience, the eye that constantly inspects and judges may follow the victim of exhaustion, even into her safe haven. It takes a lot of sleep to erase the imprint of memories that are all too present.

According to some theorists, burnout rates are higher among women simply because they are more in touch with their bodies and thus more likely to consult doctors, with the result that their experiences are more likely to be reported. This interpretation is highly specious, not only because it depends on outdated clichés to support an explanation that has nothing to do with the actual causes of the problem, but also because it fails to take into account the complexity of what Pascale Molinier aptly described as "the enigma of the working woman."[39] It is much more relevant to recognize that women in the working world today are confronted, along with their male colleagues, by the three factors we have already examined, namely, the collapse of perfectionism, the exhaustion of humanism, and the quest for recognition. But in addition, realities that are unique to the female experience, compounded by the chauvinistic atmosphere that pervades certain work environments, act as aggravating factors that reinforce each of these problems and increase the risk of overload. Women must, first of all, cope with the same difficulties that men face. The struggle to remain human in world that is becoming more and more technologized, frenetic, and complex takes a toll on members of both sexes. But women are also subject to specific pressures because the world in which they work was constructed by men and for men, in the context of an atavistic division of labor that

38 Herbert Freudenberger and Gail North, *Women's Burnout*, London, Penguin, 1985, p. 80.

39 Pascale Molinier, *L'Énigme de la femme active. Sexe, égoïsme et compassion* [*The Enigma of the Working Woman: Sex, Egoism, and Compassion*], Paris, Payot, 2003.

continues to be a source of injustice to this day. To give a concrete example, the acceleration of time, and the resulting impression of not having a single moment to oneself, is a phenomenon experienced by both genders. But for women, there are often additional, time-consuming responsibilities associated with raising children and having to adapt one's schedule to theirs. The burden of negotiating this additional set of constraints most often falls to them, as does the sense of guilt for not being able to give one's children more of one's time. It is unsurprising, therefore, that women would be more susceptible to burnout.

Working women, insists Pascale Molinier, are in no way "masculinized," nor are they channeling some masculine part of themselves:

> The working woman is, as her name suggests, both a woman and a worker. To put it another way, the new social norm of the working woman is still linked to certain traditional standards of femininity, but it is also emancipated from them. This emancipation represents more than a shift in meaning: it amounts to a revolution in our system of thought.[40]

In combination with the three principal risk factors for burnout that we have already identified, the burden of maintaining the dual identities of femininity and professionalism may well lead, in contemporary society, to moments of breathlessness.

Being perfect in a man's world

We have already seen that adapting to certain work environments can be so difficult and demand so much energy that workers no longer have time to devote to their most important pursuit: self-realization. They attempt to respond to every request, to match the ideal of the perfect employee. But in so doing, they completely neglect their own needs. This situation can prove even more difficult for women negotiating an

[40] *Ibid.*, p. 26.

environment created by men. The worldviews espoused by men, though they may be no better or worse than any others, remain resolutely masculine, and it must be acknowledged that adapting to a universe shaped by members of the opposite sex demands more effort than navigating an environment whose rules have been second nature since childhood. When Joseph Conrad wrote, in his novel *Chance*, that being a woman "is a terribly difficult task, since it consists principally in dealing with men," he might as well have been describing certain contemporary corporate environments.

The white, male engineer has been long been ensconced, in the words of Pascale Molinier, as "the standard of intelligence," but it must be conceded that he is also the source of its fatal flaw. It was he and his spiritual forefathers—Descartes, Bacon, Auguste Comte and Saint-Simon—who subjected the human mind to the great purge that stripped it of all affect and emotion, the most elemental and precious features that we typically identify with life itself. Instrumental logic, so dominant today that at this point it can only continue to evolve, is a masculine construction. Men, adds Molinier, in their dominant position, "have progressively filled the world with concrete manifestations of their abstract intelligence: numbers, ratios, diagrams, quantified measurements, complex systems, robots, rational and strategic plans, programs of action, new communication technologies."[41] The result has been the ascendance of what may be the defining characteristic of our times, the pervasive atmosphere of seriousness that envelops our planet, occasionally letting through a few sanctioned diversions that serve its purposes, but otherwise demanding that we prostrate ourselves before numbers, comply with economic dictates, and accept that life is a difficult struggle.

This austerity can be traced back to the beginnings of capitalism. It is visible, for example, at the *National Gallery* in London, in the face of

[41] *Ibid.*, p. 137. See also on this topic the analyses of Isabelle Sorrente in *Addiction générale* [*General Addiction*] (Paris, Jean-Claude Lattès, 2011), which further explores a fundamental theme developed earlier by Ernst Jünger in *Zahlen und Götter* [*Numbers and Gods*], (Stuttgart, Klett-Cotta, 1975), and by René Guénon in *Le Règne de la quantité et les signes des temps* [*The Reign of Quantity and the Signs of the Times*] (Paris, Gallimard, "NRF tradition," 1945).

the prominent Italian banker Giovanni Arnolfini, painted, with his wife, by Jan Van Eyck in 1434. The Dutch master saw through to his core. He conveyed, in those pinched, hard lips, that icy glance, that formal, self-important gesture of the hand, how cruel a man who thinks himself responsible can be, and how infectious his *ennui*. Arnolfini remains the prototype to this day for every authoritarian boss who takes pleasure in making others cower. Their power distances them from the suffering of those whose health they destroy. They seem willfully oblivious to human frailty. They present themselves as upstanding citizens, beyond reproach, sneering at the unsavory elements of life. The serious men of today remain, as they were in Van Eyck's time, conservatively dressed, prepared to venture out into the world. As for the stunning colors that Arnolfini's wife wears so beguilingly, they will remain a private fantasy. We sense that they are merely tolerated, and always kept inside the house, within sight of a blood-red bed.

And yet, these colors are the symbolic antidote to the seriousness of the masculine perspective that eschews them. Women still wear them, just as they continue to speak on behalf of values which are not now in fashion, but which humankind desperately needs: spirit, compassion, imagination. It is understandable that having to fight a battle on two fronts might sometimes leave them fatigued. For, adapting to the system isn't enough. It is also necessary to work against it, to open up spaces within it that reflect a set of perspectives as varied and rich as all of human experience. There is nothing, therefore, to be envied about the perfectionistic attitude that is so often encountered among women suffering from burnout.[42] Rather, it must be seen as the sign of an underlying problem.

This type of perfectionism can arise among women who unconsciously feel that they are "indebted" to the company that employs them, perhaps because their hiring is perceived as a token concession to gender equality. They compensate with a superhuman expenditure

42 A very interesting analysis of the behaviors of personalities at risk can be found in Michel Delbrouck's *Comment traiter le burn-out* [*How to Treat Burnout*], Brussels, De Boeck, 2011, pp. 58–60.

of effort, believing they owe it to their employer. In other cases of perfectionism, Freudenberger diagnoses a "dual mind." The sufferer wants to express herself as a woman and follow her instincts. But in the back of her mind, the voice of self-doubt urges her to trust others more than herself, and to conform to the standards set by corporate culture.[43] Unable to comply with both voices, she chooses a third option: being perfect. She imagines that this course of action will resolve her problem. She will be inimitable, since no one will be able to match her productivity, but also perfectly aligned with all standards, since she will do everything that is expected of her, and even more. Perfection seems like the only way out, a means to emerge victorious on all fronts: she will be entirely feminine, completely professional. But this solution may prove illusory, despite the interminably long days at the office and the deepening circles under her eyes. To resolve the contradiction, a more productive solution would be one that works to modify the dominant mindset, so that being a working woman becomes as unremarkable as being a working man.

The compassion trap

The exhaustion of humanism also takes on a particular significance when considered in terms of its impact on women. This second risk factor for burnout particularly affects members of the caring professions who accompany us through crucial stages in our lives: early childhood, schooling, illness, old age. Many of these professional roles are primarily filled by women. At day-care centers, kindergartens, schools, hospitals, and nursing homes, it is most often female workers who are charged with tending to the needs of others. The work they do is invaluable, yet it is often all but invisible. Our current age, which fetishizes the useful, displays considerable impatience toward those critical moments of our lives in which subtle and affective elements predominate. It is often assumed that the women who tend to us at these moments are simply drawing upon reserves of compassion with which they are innately

[43] Herbert Freudenberger, *Women's Burn-Out, op. cit.*, p. 124.

endowed. Helping, advocating for, and sharing the burdens of others are supposedly "typically feminine" behaviors. Comfortable with fragility, experienced with suffering, patient and gentle, they naturally gravitate toward positions that allow them to express these aspects of their inner nature, and it is only reasonable that men should take this into account when assigning work responsibilities.

But the presumed link between femininity and compassion is a dangerous trap that urgently needs to be dismantled, as Pascale Molinier makes clear. Compassion is not some inborn, immutable feature like hair color. Caring for others' well-being is more of a "social construct . . . the result of a collaborative effort"[44] with its own codes, requirements, difficulties and pleasures. Schopenhauer attributed the capacity for justice to men, and the capacity for charity to women. It must be noted that for all of his merits as a philosopher, he was a miserable human being who never showed respect to anyone other than his dog. There is truly no fainter praise with which to damn a person than to bestow upon her the title of "charitable by nature." This label, in fact, ensures that any problems that arise will be chalked up to her feminine temperament, which is falsely assumed to be overflowing with excesses of human kindness. In cases of overwork, like that of the nurses shadowed by Pascale Molinier, who themselves self-identified as "extremists of the extreme," their failure to stay on top of everything is automatically attributed to a flaw in their character. They are told: "it's because you're too invested, it's in your nature, you're too devoted, stop getting carried away . . ." And, in this way, their opinions "are frequently overruled or disregarded on the grounds of personal instability."[45]

There is no conclusive evidence that their problems stem from a surfeit of compassion. They are more likely the result of understaffing or inefficient organization of the workforce. Yet, the association between femininity and concern for others is so entrenched that it is often invoked as an explanatory factor:

[44] Pascale Molinier, *L'Énigme de la femme active* [*The Enigma of the Working Woman*], *op. cit.*, p. 11.

[45] *Ibid.*, p. 192.

> All women are supposed to possess that famous "relational self" transmitted from mother to daughter, to be further honed by the experience of motherhood … Lapses of empathy are viewed as a corruption of femininity.[46]

By this point, the trap is dangerously close to snapping shut, for in many cases, the worker saddled with these assumptions cannot help but sink into self-recrimination, assuming that any problems that arise are the result of her own personal failings—not only as an employee, but more damningly, as a woman—when in reality, they stem from circumstances external to her. When a nursery school instructor finds herself overwhelmed by ten screaming children, it most likely has nothing to do with her gender, and everything to do with insufficient staffing. Yet burnout, here labeled "compassion overload"[47] because it signals the breakdown of nurturing behaviors, will almost inevitably be attributed to internal factors. In this climate, we see nurses apologizing for falling short of expectations or not being able to "keep it together." The problems are thus "psychologized": these women comb through their personal histories, searching for the causes of their failures, instead of analyzing the social conditions of their work environments and looking for ways to improve them. Compassion, always a precious virtue, is in this context a professional attribute; it should be treated as such, and not as some vaguely magical sensitivity that allows its possessor to work miracles under extreme conditions. Only in this way can it be appreciated for what it is, as one of the most visible ways of "pursuing happiness, in a world where suffering has not been forgotten."[48]

Recognition and motherhood

We have already identified the quest for recognition as a third factor accounting for certain cases of burnout. Men and women have both been known peer into the eyes of others, searching for some indication

46 *Ibid.*, p. 87.
47 *Ibid.*, p. 190.
48 *Ibid.*, p. 117.

that their efforts have not been in vain. They want confirmation that they are valuable. In a complex world, the competition for this confirmation is so fierce that there never seems to be quite enough recognition to go around.

But here too, the problems that are so characteristic of our times are intensified for women, because, for the mothers among them, there is one group of people who can provide them with a type of recognition unlike any other: their children. In our attempts to distribute our limited resources among the people who lay claim to them, our children are, so to speak, in a class by themselves. They are an absolute, not just as human beings, but as the flesh of our flesh, the product of our desires, to whom we have promised a liberated future that will be all the more beautiful if only we can lead them to it. The experience of motherhood, largely neglected by philosophers over the course of history, is one of the most awe-inspiring of all life events. It perpetuates a biological miracle that has been repeating itself since the dawn of our species and a practice that can scarcely be taught or learned, but which nonetheless has the capacity to transform a destiny: the act of raising a child. The mystery of being human—and it is, indeed, a mystery—suddenly solidifies into the shape of a small child, who fixes the world with a penetrating gaze. And that gaze often lands upon a mother whose presence is a source of comfort, but whose attention is also a resource to be monopolized. It is the start of a story that promises, above all, to be unpredictable.

For a woman, this birth changes everything. But, beyond the grace period of those first few months, life continues on essentially as it had before. There are still the same emails to be answered, the same professional obligations to be met—to be a good network engineer, an effective police officer, or an enthusiastic professor. This tiny change has scarcely stopped the world from turning. And yet, from a certain point of view, it is no longer turning in quite the same way, as if a new magnetic field were interfering with the forces that previously guided it, subtly shifting its trajectory in space.

In this tension between "everything is different" and "everything is the same," a balance must be struck, even as the question of recognition is upended by it. Before, the goal was to be a competent professional and an appealing partner or spouse. But now, in addition, there is the desire to be recognized as a good mother. This supplementary responsibility cannot simply be added on to all the pre-existing roles that must be filled. It is something separate, a new category of its own: an exception must be made for motherhood.

This only further complicates the situation. Working women today are navigating problems so new that we do not yet have sufficient distance to evaluate them. The challenges they face range from determining the implications of stem cell research to trying to stay true to themselves while managing an all-male team. And alongside these new and difficult challenges, there remains the age-old pressure to be a "good mother," an expectation that drags with it not only the baggage specific to each individual family, but also the Christian archetypes of the *mater dolorosa* and the mother of God, the strength and the stereotypes associated with Jewish mothers, the spirits of matriarchal leaders, the specter of castration anxiety, and a host of other images, conscious or unconscious, that permeate the psyche, connecting it to an ancient practice that is always beginning anew and always different. There is a striking clash, here, between two different worlds. On one side is the modern conception of the working woman, equal to men in all respects. On the other side is an initiation into that strange mixture of biology and tradition which has always been a part of the human experience. And when this collision of worlds is taking place against a backdrop of crying babies, toddler tantrums, sleepless nights, financial difficulties, problems at school, and domestic squabbles, it's not hard to understand how a certain amount of fatigue might result.

Violaine Guéricault has written about the phenomenon of maternal burnout.[49] This is a dimension of burnout that should not be underestimated—that might, in fact, be critical. Many writings about burnout only take into account the professional conditions that incite fatigue, as though family life could never contribute to exhaustion. In

49 Violaine Guéricault, *La Fatigue émotionnelle et physique des mères* [*The Physical and Emotional Fatigue of Mothers*], Paris, Odile Jacob, 2004.

reality, it seems to play a decisive role in many cases, even if it is not the principal cause. Burnout is a disorder caused by excess. Its current prevalence is a reflection of the mounting pressures that affect all sectors of modern society. For the working woman who chooses to become a mother, this excess is compounded by the merging of what were considered, only a few decades ago, to be two separate, full-time occupations. Recent experience demonstrates that an evolution in prevalent attitudes—especially among men—and adjustments to the socio-economic conditions of the working world are urgently needed, if working women are to be granted, quite simply, the time to live their lives.

Part III

Postmodern Malaise

Theory of a mirror disorder

Included among the pathologies of civilization are the various types of ill-defined *malaise* experienced by certain individuals as a response to social conditions they cannot tolerate. It matters little whether those afflicted are inveterate contrarians or, on the contrary, faithful representatives of the status quo. What matters is that they experience an episode of secession from their situation. Their state of mind reflects the dysfunctionality of the system to which they belong, and the form that their renunciation takes is influenced by the values to which they had previously subscribed. Such diseases of civilization are, in essence, mirror disorders, reflecting the aspects of a society that are accepted with the greatest difficulty.

Burnout is the current name for this type of condition. An illness that arises as a response to excess, overload, stress, loss of meaning, the dictates of the profit motive, and the strain of upholding humanist values within a technocratic system, it reveals the darker aspects of modern corporate culture. In this respect, it is more a reactive disorder than an endogenous illness: its causes are often external to the individual, originating from his or her interactions with a professional environment.

A secret, shared lineage connects all the symptoms of malaise induced by civilization, just as it unites the sensitive people from every age in history who longed to see their contemporaries behave with more reason and dignity. Condemnation of the system is the hallmark of those states of mind in which the individual concludes—after careful consideration and a certain amount of soul-searching—that while he or she may not be beyond reproach, the world, for its part, deserves to be judged critically. In order to express such malaise, new language was created. Often, this was as much a matter of self-preservation as it was self-expression: artistic and intellectual pursuits have always provided an outlet and a refuge for those enlightened souls who might otherwise have turned to self-destruction. New words were coined, each bearing the imprint of the era that gave rise to it, since mirror disorders, by their very nature, must be historically specific, functioning as a way for those afflicted to gain distance from a particular situation. It is important to trace the history of these maladies of civilization and to situate burnout within a modern tradition of expressions of dissent, in order to recognize it in its postmodern form.

Acedia, as we have already discussed, was a way of seceding from monastic life, its constraints, and the fate it reserved for those who doubted its tenets. The condition endured beyond its ecclesiastical incarnation, but in the course of this transformation, it was bestowed with a new name. It became *spleen*, in the Baudelairean sense. The affective states that characterize both conditions are essentially the same: sadness, *ennui*, hopelessness and melancholy seem to traverse time, more or less unchanged. In a little-known essay, Aldous Huxley explicitly identifies the *ennui* of the nineteenth century as a direct descendant of the acedia experienced by monks:

> It is a very curious phenomenon, this progress of accidie [*sic*] from the position of being a deadly sin, deserving of damnation, to the position first of a disease and finally of an essentially lyrical emotion, fruitful in the inspiration of much of the most characteristic modern literature.[1]

Acedia has, in fact, passed through several phases in the course of its metamorphosis, renamed "melancholy," then "spleen," then "ennui" and "neurasthenia." But through all of these transformations, its function as a form of protest remained intact.

1 Aldous Huxley, "Accidie," in *On the Margin*, London, Chatto & Windus, 1923, p. 22. He also writes: "accidie is still with us as an inspiration, one of the most serious and poignant of literary themes" (p. 23).

Baudelaire's was an especially severe case. He himself makes the distinction between the universal aspects of his condition and those that he ascribed to the new iron age in which he saw the last of his ideals going to ruin. His spleen has a meta-historical component, comprising damnation and the desire for redemption, original sin and the determination to bring into being a Beauty—forged from an amalgam of art and life—that would outshine the surrounding decay. When, in *Les plaintes d'un Icare* (*The Complaints of an Icarus*), he explains that he, too, has burned his wings "sous je ne sais quel oeil de feu" ("under I know not what fiery eye") and that his own scorched eyes "ne voient que des souvenirs de soleil" ("see only memories of sun"),[2] the theme he evokes is a timeless one. The problem of his "déménagement" ("relocation"), which he endlessly discusses with his soul, cannot be resolved by a voyage to Lisbon, Holland, or even Tornio. He must go "n'importe où! n'importe où! pourvu que ce soit hors de ce monde" ("Anywhere! As long as it is out of the world").[3] Here, too, his yearning belongs to every age, and to every deserter eternally on the run. His desertion is metaphysical. Nonetheless, the "je ne veux pas" ("I will not") that he snarls at the end of *Rebelle* (*Rebel*), and which he was to abbreviate—after a peculiar set of circumstances brought him to Brussels at the end of his life—to an implacable "Crénom!,"[4] also resonates as the rejection of a particular reality, that of France in the 1860s. "Je veux dater ma colère" ("I want to put a date to my anger"), he writes in *Fusées*.[5] His spleen becomes the primary evidence in the case he levies against modernity, progress and mechanization. For Baudelaire, the era itself must be found guilty of making man's exile from the "vert paradis des amours enfantines" ("green paradise of childish loves") ever more definitive and irremediable. Progress, that "doctrine de paresseux,

2 Charles Baudelaire, *Les Fleurs du Mal*, Paris, Gallimard, 1972, p. 221.

3 Charles Baudelaire, *Le Spleen de Paris*, Paris, Flammarion, 1987, p. 178.

4 Translator's note: Near the end of his life, Baudelaire left Paris for Brussels, where he suffered a massive stroke that left him semi-paralyzed and aphasic. The only word he was able to speak in the months before his death was the expletive "Crénom," roughly equivalent to "Goddamn!"

5 Charles Baudelaire, *Fusées*, Paris, Gallimard, 1986, p. 85.

doctrine de Belges" ("doctrine of idlers, doctrine of the Belgians"),[6] rids the earth of its last memories of heroism. All that remains is nostalgia for a Golden Age, the last fantastic traces of which are to be permanently erased by an industrialized civilization.

A decade later, it was neurasthenia that preoccupied European literature. From the end of the nineteenth century until World War I, it served as the banner beneath which individual symptoms, including fatigue, anxiety, headache and depression, were grouped together with a socio-political prognosis. In the writings of Proust, or in Thomas Mann's *Magic Mountain*, neurasthenia and its derivatives allowed for a dissenting discourse concerning the ideology of the era. Allegedly American in origin, it was the price that certain contemplative minds had to pay to a society they judged too restless, facile and materialistic. The primary target was still progress and the modern organization of the working world—for example, in the writings of Virginia Woolf, whom we can imagine heaving a deep sigh amidst the mechanical din of the industrial revolution. It was with a sense of resignation in the face of the inevitable that she wrote: "A million hands stitch, raise hods with bricks. The activity is endless. And tomorrow it begins again . . ."[7]

The succession of pathologies of civilization appears, at first glance, to be interrupted after World War I. From this point on, paranoia and then schizophrenia occupy a central place in literature and philosophy, but unlike acedia, spleen, or neurasthenia, they were not seen as mirror disorders by many writers, whose views would later be contested, notably by Deleuze and Guattari. These two severe psychoses—paranoia and schizophrenia—were classified instead as opaque disorders, with endogenous causes. For this reason, some researchers have suggested, it would seem inappropriate to link them to a socio-political agenda. Their relatively even distribution across populations, time periods, and geographic locations seems to preclude an interpretation that characterizes them as reactions to a particular historical period or situation.

[6] Charles Baudelaire, *Mon coeur mis à nu*, Paris, Gallimard, 1986, p. 95.

[7] V. Woolf, *The Waves*, Oxford University Press, 1992, p. 103.

Despite these fundamental difficulties, both of these psychoses have, in fact, taken on the function of mirror disorders, in the hands of writers and philosophers who used them to expose the unsavory realities of the times in which they wrote. A number of novelists have turned to evocations of paranoia in an effort to convey the effect that totalitarian societies have on individuals. Kafka in *The Trial*, Huxley in *Brave New World* and Orwell in *1984*, portray pathetic heroes crushed by the machinations of anonymous organizations whose cruelty is ideological. The affliction from which they sufferer does not originate within the mind of the individual; it is a reaction to a political system that deliberately incites terror on a global scale as a means to control bodies and minds. More recently, in their book entitled *Anti-Oedipus*, Gilles Deleuze and Félix Guattari have used schizophrenia to present a political prognosis for an information-based society where everything has become flux, a matter of encoding and decoding. The book's subtitle, "*Capitalism and Schizophrenia*," clearly puts forward their premise that the mental disorder and the political system in question function as reflections of one another. "Schizophrenia as a process" they write, "is desiring-production ... It is our very own 'malady,' modern man's sickness."[8] This politicization of a devastating mental illness could be seen as offensive, and understandably so. But that concern is somewhat alleviated if we interpret it—though the authors themselves might not agree with this interpretation—as an illuminating metaphor for the philosophy of desire for which the events of May 1968 sounded the fanfare.

As for depression, it cannot be classified as a disease of civilization. It is less like a mirror and more like a bottomless pit, reflecting nothing, letting in no light. For this reason, it must be characterized as an opaque disorder, distinct from burnout. To be sure, a severe case of burnout

[8] G. Deleuze and F. Guattari, *Anti-Oedipus*, trans. Robert Hurley, Mark Seem, and Helen R. Lane, London, Viking, 1984, p. 142. There is no better illustration of the liberties taken by the authors with regards to this "malady" than the following bit of bravado: "We are still too competent; we would like to speak in the name of an absolute incompetence. Someone asked us if we had ever seen a schizophrenic—no, no, we have never seen one" (p. 380).

may lead to a depressive state, and we would be ill-advised to insist on excessively clear-cut delineations where mental disorders are concerned. Nonetheless, there are several key differences that separate these two conditions. Michel Delbrouck highlights the most important one:

> In burnout, initially, only one's professional life is affected, whereas, in depression, the loss of interest and the inability to experience pleasure (anhedonia) extend to all spheres of life, including family, friendships, leisure, etc."[9]

Depression may strike anyone, anywhere, whereas burnout is inherently tied to a professional context. Depression is thus more difficult to explain or comprehend. In his extraordinary essay on the topic, William Styron insists upon "the basic inability of healthy people to imagine a form of torment so alien to everyday experience."[10] He also emphasizes, in this collection of pages where every word resonates with sincerity and courage, the "ferocious *inwardness* of the pain"[11] that a biochemical abnormality of the brain can elicit. The acute sense of loss, guilt, and self-loathing that occur in cases of depression do not manifest with the same intensity in cases of burnout.

Depression is not, therefore, a mirror disorder, reflecting back certain characteristics of the external system in which it arises. It is, instead, a place of darkness and despondency that those afflicted must pass through, and from which, if they are fortunate, they may emerge, like William Styron at the end of his essay, echoing the final words of Dante's *Inferno*: "E quindi uscimmo a riveder le stelle." ("And so we came forth, and once again beheld the stars.") If, somehow, from the depths of its opacity, we were to extract a meaning that mirrors certain aspects of reality, the truth reflected there would have to be a universal one. Styron is among those who conceive of depression in this way:

9 Michel Delbrouck, *Comment traiter le burn-out* [*How to Treat Burnout*], *op. cit.*, p. 36. To further emphasize this difference between burnout and depression, we might note that in his thoroughly researched book on the latter topic, *The Noonday Demon: An Atlas of Depression* (New York, Simon and Schuster, 2001), Andrew Solomon makes no mention of burnout or of the working world, as if they occupied a completely different universe.

10 William Styron, *Darkness Visible: A Memoir of Madness*, *op. cit.*, p. 17.

11 *Ibid.*, p. 20.

> But in science and art the search will doubtless go on for a clear representation of its meaning, which sometimes, for those who have known it, is a simulacrum of all the evil of our world: of our everyday discord and chaos, our irrationality, warfare and crime, torture and violence, our impulse toward death and our flight from it held in the intolerable equipoise of history.[12]

These images transcend time and geography; they are common to every age in history and to every continent on the planet.

The expression "pathology of civilization" is problematic, in any case, in that it downplays the singularity of each individual's experience of mental illness and the unique biochemical processes of the brain that give rise to it. As such, it must be no more than the complement to the kind of individualized analysis that medicine and psychopathology can provide. Another ambiguity of the expression is that it may be interpreted to mean either that civilization itself is diseased, or that the illness in question is a product of civilization. In the first case, the emphasis is placed on society, and in the second, on the individual. Sociologists might say that society is filtered through individual psyches, while psychologists would maintain that individuals struggle to integrate external pressures.

There is truth in both of these perspectives, but the philosophical approach brings with it a third point of view. It asks us to consider what is happening in the middle, in the *relationship* between the individual and society. These two entities evolve conjointly: everything happens in the interactions between them. If we agree to look at things in this way, the expression "pathology of civilization" takes on a more precise meaning: it describes a dysfunctional relationship. The fault does not lie solely with the individual sufferers. Neither their cerebral function, nor the state of their psychological landscape can account for everything. And conversely, it would be excessive to lay all the blame on the abstract entity that is society.

In an article on the connections between work and sexuality, Christophe Dejours offers an insightful way of framing the dilemma. In

12 *Ibid.*, p. 83.

one view, he explains, society is perceived as "a selfish and destructive giant." We ascribe to it "a colossal amount of power, dwarfing that of our unconscious desires."[13] It is capable of coercion, of imposing its will upon us, to the point of inflicting psychological torture. It is a locus of power, pathogenic at every level, and the individual who confronts it is reduced to the position of a "defenseless child, bereft of resources." It is within this model, notes Dejours, that we most often hear talk of stress and aggression. As for the other model, it seems to err in the opposite direction, depicting society as relatively neutral: "it is what it is and it's the same for everyone." The implication is that society cannot be the source of the problem, because if it were, all of its members would be equally affected. The original trauma must therefore be traced back to the afflicted individuals—to their weaknesses, their neuroses, and their inner conflicts. Even if the trouble first surfaces in the context of a work environment, we need not look to this environment for an explanation. We would do better to turn our attentions to the personal history of the subject, rather than his or her working conditions. Dejours concludes his comparison with these words:

> Each approach has its merits, even if neither allows us to conclusively determine whether it is society or the individual that is responsible for the suffering and ill health of those who work (and those who do not).[14]

At first glance, there seems to be no good solution for this epistemological problem. We could pick a side and assign responsibility to a single factor. Such a theory could be described as "vectorial": it purports to identify the source of the problem, to discriminate between cause and effect. Alternatively, we could choose not to choose, acknowledging that only a multifactorial analysis could do justice to the complexity of the situation. Undoubtedly, there is more intellectual honesty in this latter

[13] Dejours, Christophe, "'Centralité du travail' et théorie de la sexualité" ["'Centrality of Work' and a theory of sexuality," in Ch. Dejours (ed.), *Observations cliniques en psychopathologie du travail* [*Clinical and Psychopathological Observations of Work*], Paris, PUF, 2010, p. 86.

[14] *Ibid.*, p. 87.

position, but on occasion, we might wish for a clearer distribution of responsibility. It is in such cases that the "relational" approach favored by philosophical inquiry enriches the debate. According to this view, in mirror disorders and diseases of civilization, it is the relationship between the individual and society that is the source of the problem. And, after all, it takes two to make a relationship.

A relationship disorder is a conflict between two entities whose respective identities are, to a large extent, overlapping and deeply intertwined. It is telling that, in most cases of burnout, the relationship that connects the individual to work, and to societal values, is extremely tight-knit. This problem does not afflict confirmed iconoclasts or anarchists—although its victims may be anarchists in the making. On the contrary, it affects well-adjusted people who work, have families, and subscribe to the established value systems. These individuals love, or seem to love, the society to which they have devoted so much energy. They are good students, hard-working and highly motivated. The psycho-social relationship is strong: these are people convinced that the key to self-fulfillment is social and professional success, who believe just as sincerely that society has need of them. It looks like the perfect relationship. But the puzzle is that this relationship nonetheless breaks down, like the bond between two lovers who look like the poster children for happiness, but who somehow wind up miserable, sleeping in separate beds.

Under the sign of fire

In this postmodern era, the sign of fire is ascendant, shaping the relationship between the individual and the world. Heirs to Prometheus, who stole fire from the gods by hiding the embers in the hollow of an elder tree, the children of the technological age have incorporated combustion into every one of their activities. It transforms matter by burning oil, igniting gas or coal, splitting the atom, or heating metals to produce light. Electricity, electronics, and the transmission of radio waves rely on energetic phenomena whose common origin is the modulation of a heat source. Greenhouse gasses, pollution, and global warming stem from the quantities of energy released by combustion reactions all over the planet.

Ours is truly a civilization born of fire. It is the only element that we have not defiled, in contrast to our pollution of water, air, and earth. Environmentalists persistently advocate for the protection of these three threatened elements, even as they wage campaigns against the various modern manifestations of incandescence. Those who "think green" valorize earth, air, and water while warning against the destructive power of fire. They are right to perceive that the determination to derive maximum benefit from the harnessing of smoke and fire is a defining a characteristic of our technological age. While air, earth, and water are persistently degraded, fire reigns supreme. It burns whatever we give it to burn; it consumes the earth's fossil layers to fuel engines and computers. Its voracity is such that it must be constantly supplied with new material to burn.

One of these new combustibles is the human psyche. It has been said that the only certain things in this world are coincidences.[15] The particular coincidence that connects burnout to the fire-centric society in which it appears is striking. Combustion is the driving force for both. Freudenberger, as we have seen, compares the burnout victim to the burned out shell of a fire-ravaged building. He returns to the same metaphor to describe the possibilities for healing: "In every fire," he writes, "even a burnt-out one, there are glowing embers. You can use them to rekindle the spark."[16] Everywhere, fire dominates.

In using the expression "burnout," Freudenberger is engaging with a very old tradition, even as he turns it on its head. His claim is that our inner fire, hitherto a sacred source of power that allowed human beings

[15] Translator's note: This is a reference to a famous quotation from the Italian writer Leonardo Sciascia: "Io credo che le sole cose sicure in questo mondo siano le coincidenze." ["I believe that the only certain things in this world are coincidences."]

[16] Freudenberger, *op. cit.*, p. xxii.

to push beyond their limits, can transform into a force of destruction. This shift in meaning testifies to the rupture that marks the start of postmodern life.

Traditionally, in fact, inner fire was the province of the privileged few. It was the secret source of their passion and their power, permitting the purification and subsequent illumination of those who were open to God's spirit. In *The Divine Comedy*, this inner fire remains the prerogative of the blessed. It is in the Empyrean, the celestial realm of pure light where God reigns and where those closest to Him abide, that the angels form nine circles of fire. Of course, the damned in Dante's vision are also subjected to a fiery ordeal, but theirs is an external conflagration: a rain of fire for those who committed violence against nature and sparks of flame for those who committed violence against art. Buddhism also speaks of an inner fire as a "penetrating consciousness, an illumination" that leads to the destruction of the outer shell: "I fan the flame within me," we read in the *Samyutta Nikaya*. "My heart is the hearth, the flame is the mastered self."[17] The inner fire is valorized, while the external fire, the fiery accident or punishment, inspires fear. In burnout, on the contrary, the inner fire is implicated in the very name of the disorder. This constitutes a radical change.

Fire is the ultimate contradiction, "the spirit that always denies," as Goethe's Mephistopheles describes himself to Faust. It is that which it is not; it varies infinitely with each of its metamorphoses. In his *Psychoanalysis of Fire*, Gaston Bachelard offers a dreamlike meditation on the many faces of fire worship. A symbol of change, its moral connotations are multiple:

> Of all natural phenomena, fire is truly the only one that effortlessly embodies either of two opposing values: good and evil. It shines in Paradise. It burns in Hell. It is comfort and torture. It is the warmth of the oven and the flames of the apocalypse. It is a pleasure for the

[17] *Symyuttanikâya* (*sic.*), 1, 169, cited by J. Chevalier and A. Gheerbrant, *Dictionnaire des symbols* [*Dictionary of Symbols*], Paris, Robert Laffont, 1982, p. 435.

> well-behaved child who sits by the hearth, but it punishes the disobedience of those who draw too close to its flames.[18]

It sets the mind alight, sparking great ideas or kindling the enthusiasm of an engaging personality who always exudes warmth and zeal. It is the inner fire that warms us and gives us energy. It is the flame that fires the soul, the source of spiritual excitation, the center of a sometimes cosmic desire. It stirs a yearning for change, a desire to speed time forward, to bring our lives to a state of heightened illumination. There is grandeur in fire, but danger also, for its dialectical nature allows it to mutate rapidly into its opposite. To burn is to be in a state of contradiction. Passion warms, but it can also scald. A flash of light illuminates the darkness, but too much light is blinding.

> As soon as a sentiment rises to the tonality of fire, as soon as it is exposed in all of its violence, the metaphysics of fire guarantee that it will accumulate a mass of contradictions.[19]

And so, inevitably, the intensity diminishes. The sensation of burning is transformed into its opposite: what had been white-hot grows cold, flat, listless, lacking fire. Fire is the element of painful ambiguities.

It is this ambivalence that manifests in cases of burnout: the inner fire, which was once the divine heat of the enthusiast, has become a psychiatric concern. The problem is that this warmth no longer has an outlet for its own expression: the technological system that now wields global influence is, in fact, the exact opposite of an inner fire. The first word that comes to mind to describe the affective tonality of this system is "cold." Instrumental reason was developed far from the warmth of the emotions. It is a product of icy precision.

A recent play by the German dramatist Falk Richter explores the world of consultants and the fate they reserve for one of their colleagues—older, ill-adapted, oversensitive, soon to be fired. The play's title, *Unter Eis* (*Under Ice*), is another reference to this system, evoked in the first scene

[18] G. Bachelard, *Psychanalyse du feu*, Paris, Gallimard, 1949, p. 24. Published in English as *Psychoanalysis of Fire* (trans. Alan C.M. Ross), Boston, Beacon Press, 1964.

[19] *Ibid.*, p. 190.

in an incantatory manner: "Frozen solid under the ice ... cold ... everything's covered in ice, nothing moves, it's all still, the shock of the cold, frozen cold, deep frozen."[20] With hard, cold precision, the characters intone the truths by which they operate, composed of numbers, certainties, economic logic, pure theory, unwavering motivation, and implacable consistency. Meanwhile, the hapless hero, Paul Niemand (Paul Nobody)—"too old to start again, too young to retire"[21]—sinks into solitude, shattered by a mentality devoid of all warmth. In this exaggerated depiction of a real phenomenon, Falk Richter gets to the heart of the matter. Some people cannot live under ice. Subjected to such pitiless dictates, they break down. Their inner fire, the manifestation of their deepest aspirations, turns against them, having been held in check for too long. It's a total blackout, says Richter.

The paradox of our modern society is that it actually purports to value enthusiasm. The desire to stoke one's inner fire, to experience the kind of exaltation that raises human beings to a superhuman level, is so widespread as to be featured on the "Health" pages of magazines. Heroism has become a collective effort, in contrast to earlier times, when Icarus fell alone. Until recently, the chance to burn one's wings was reserved for a few exceptional individuals, a handful of demigods who managed to escape the fate of ordinary mortals, willing to pay the ultimate price in exchange for an exceptional destiny. Flying so close to the sun could only be the act of a tragic hero. This is the message conveyed by the most beautiful, but also the least truthful, of the Breughel paintings on view at the Royal Museums of Fine Arts in Brussels: *Landscape with the Fall of Icarus*. The eponymous hero has fallen alone, and is drowning alone in a corner of the painting. His cries have not resonated. No one has heard him calling to his distant father. His fall has been met with indifference. Only a few floating feathers

20 Falk Richter (trans. David Tushingham) *Under Ice*, S. Fischer Verlag, 2004, p. 5.

21 *Ibid.*, p. 7. In his excellent novel *La Question Humaine* [*The Human Question*], which also takes place in a corporate milieu, François Emmanuel speaks of a "frozen madness" with regard to his protagonist, a madness kept under ice that is soon unleashed to burn unchecked (Paris, Stock, 2000, p. 71).

silently bear witness to the drama that has taken place. The fisherman sitting nearby has not allowed himself to be distracted by the plunging figure of this giant man-bird. In the foreground, the ploughman with the wide, red sleeves remains unperturbed. The shepherd is looking elsewhere, preoccupied with some mundane concern, oblivious to the drama that the sun setting behind him has wrought. The lesson to be gleaned from Breughel, which is absent from the Ovidian account that inspired him, is that it is better to tend to one's own affairs and let the madmen burn their wings. This piece of wisdom upholds indifference and detachment as positive values, just as the Neostoic movement did in Renaissance times. The heroes alone will suffer for their excesses. Their overheated ambitions are of no interest to the little people in the fields or on the shore.

But, now that burning one's wings is a matter that concerns our entire society—to the point that the associated pathologies are sometimes covered by health insurance—indifference is no longer permitted. Excess is no longer the folly of isolated individuals. It is collective. Burning one's wings due to excessive striving has become mundane. Flying too close to the sun—represented by power and wealth—or even simply participating in an overheated system, leads many people to a state of fatigue that sends them into freefall. Icarus is no longer alone. It is as if our entire society were determined to fly as close as possible to some nameless sun, no matter what the price.

But what sun is this? And what is this undertaking? Is it the verticality that Sloterdijk describes in his great book *You Must Change Your Life*, where he attempts to spark "the holy fire of exaggeration"[22] in an era of emotional numbness whose greatest achievements revolve around consumption and production? The ascetics, the saints, the sages, the philosophers, the artists and the virtuosos, those who made a profession of exposing themselves to the risks of overheating, the dangers of madness and delirium, have lost their monopoly on excess. Those on

[22] P. Sloterdijk (trans. Wieland Hoban), *You Must Change Your Life*, Cambridge, Polity Press, 2013, p. 403.

whom the burdens of the human condition had previously rested have seen themselves outdone by far more virulent sources of power. And yet, they alone have the potential to guide us in a new direction.

Burnout, that incandescence of the system that turns against itself, is the affliction of our times. And the same affliction that has befallen a portion of its population is ravaging our equally exhausted Earth. Burnout is an imbalance. It is only by seeking a way to regain our equilibrium, on both a personal and societal level, that we can find a viable path forward.

The tightrope-walker's manifesto

By now, this investigation into the nature of burnout may have left the reader feeling somewhat discouraged about the capacity of language to effect meaningful change. Indeed, faced with the complexities of modern life, the philosopher's customary toolkit of words and concepts begins to look suspiciously inadequate. Who would believe that thought alone could counteract the excesses that a potent combination of technology, economics, and demographics have given rise to? Technological systems are constantly expanding, profit-hungry investors demand ever-increasing returns, and every day, a fresh batch of consumers enters the global marketplace. The current system thrives on maximization: more things, more money, more interactions, more distractions. This is the nature of our reality, and when measured against the capitalistic logic that drives it, philosophical pursuits may appear laughably ineffectual.

"Humankind loves the dramatic," as Bergson said, and the frenetic logic that holds us under its spell seems destined to retain that hold for many years to come. It is entirely possible that in twenty years, the combined effects of economic deregulation and global competition will have rendered commonplace certain managerial techniques that today strike us as unbearably harsh. And this may, in turn, be no more than a prelude to still more violent pressures exerted on the working world by ever more efficient instruments of control. The seeds have already been sewn, and surely a handful of words will not uproot them, not when they are nurtured by the logic of anonymous systems and structures.

If things were clearer, at least, we might have combat instead of burnout. The enemies would be identifiable, and blame could be more easily assigned. But the postmodern age, like every other interesting period in human history, is characterized by the most intense ambiguity. It resists Manichean classifications; a categorical condemnation of our technological and economic systems would be the least credible response to this disease of civilization. In fact, the ascendance of these systems directly accounts for some of the most admirable aspects of the world as we know it. Technology, in its synthesis of nature and intelligence, exemplified by modern advancements in medical treatment, has taken the utopian visions of our ancient ancestors and made them real. Economic development is the driving force in the fight to end poverty, which has brought greater dignity to the lives of many. It would be an error of oversimplification to insist that our tools and our wealth had given us nothing but sickness and misery; on the contrary, as the global population rapidly approaches eight billion, they are more essential to humankind than ever before. What is at issue is not the systems themselves, but rather the excesses that drive their development. This is why the ambiguity of our current situation remains intractable.

What, then, can philosophers do, with their books and their abstract concepts? How can they overcome an overwhelming sense of discouragement? Like anyone recovering from burnout, they must refocus their objectives on that which is most important to them and remain faithful to it. For "*revivre* (to live again),"[23] as Frédéric Worms describes it, must surely still be possible, if only we can find a way to change and, in so doing, to rid ourselves of the harmful beliefs and pressures that weigh upon us. A certain amount of egoism can sometimes be healthy. We would also do well to heed Deleuze's admonition to flee

[23] Frédéric Worms, *Revivre*, Paris, Flammarion, 2012.

courageously,[24] even if, in our flight, we never get farther than recreating, somewhere else, an environment that gives us the tranquility to express our own desires. In this sense, a "successful" burnout, if we may be permitted this seemingly oxymoronic expression, is one that culminates in a metamorphosis. The individual reconnects with the things that hold meaning for her, in what we must assume is a happy reunion.

This notion of staying true to oneself also applies to philosophy. Even if the concept remains a fragile one, even if it is already the ostensible focus of all contemporary thought, philosophers must continue to consider what a better life might look like. It would be an appalling waste if the era that has enjoyed the greatest material gains were also to be the most impoverished in terms of meaning and spirituality. For this reason, any ideas that point us toward reconstruction, however small in scale, acquire a sense of urgency.

Two concepts in particular seem indispensable here: that of balance and that of a pact.

What is equilibrium, if not the capacity to be thrown off balance without falling? Balance is like time: we know what it is, but we struggle to define it. We only begin to ponder its meaning when it is absent. We never consider the strange miracle that is the ability to walk until we find ourselves with a broken leg. That's when the questions start. And the more we think about it, the more it seems improbable that anyone could manage to remain upright, supported only by a platform as narrow as the sole of a human foot.

In the same way, when a person's sense of balance is broken, to the point where catching the train to work begins to feel like an insurmountable task, questions abruptly arise. What previously went without saying suddenly becomes a problem. Dedicating one's life to a corporation no longer seems like a reasonable decision; adhering to the demands of a ridiculous schedule no longer feels sustainable. But how can we find a new state of balance, when we arrived at the previous one

24 Translator's note: See *Anti-Oedipus* (*op. cit.*), p. 374: "Courage consists . . . in agreeing to flee rather than live tranquilly and hypocritically in false refuges."

without even thinking about it, when working once came as naturally as walking? And how can we maintain or new-found equilibrium in a society that remains unchanged? These are the questions we face as we negotiate life after burnout.

As human beings, we are obliged to reconcile two types of balance that often wind up at odds with one another. The first is *intuitive equilibrium*. Its focus is the body, always seeking a happy medium, an ideal balance between too much and too little sleep, food, or activity. Except in certain specific contexts, the body shies away from extremes, avoiding compulsive excesses and steering clear of obsessional exertions. This personal sense of harmony is guided by intuition, which differs for each individual: some are highly attuned to the messages their bodies send them, while others register only the strongest signals. In our society, where the physical self is often barely acknowledged, reconnecting with the body's intuitive equilibrium—through yoga, sport, or relaxation—can be highly beneficial.

Life would be a paradise if this were the only type of equilibrium we had to reckon with. To be happy, we would need only to listen to our inner selves, to exercise our bodies and frequent the baths, like the ancient Greeks, who, for their part, never seemed far from a state of happiness. It was to celebrate this happiness, and to demonstrate that it lay within man's reach, that they invented philosophy. But living is more complicated than that, for we must also contend with *normative equilibrium*. In order to function within a society, our personal intuitions must yield to collective norms. These norms also seek to establish a kind of equilibrium, but, in this case, the guiding principle is not attunement to one's inner self, but rather obedience to laws set in place by others. The fact that this normative equilibrium is externally dictated, and often imposed upon the individual, leaves it open to contestation. While it is sometimes presented as "natural," normative equilibrium is, in reality, purely a social construct and, as such, it can take a wide variety of forms. If it does not result from a genuinely democratic deliberation process, it cannot legitimately claim to regulate an individual's intuitive equilibrium, and this is why it so often meets with resistance.

The ancient view of society as a single, vast organism, attests to a sense of continuity between the intuitive and the normative, at least on a metaphorical level. In this ideal configuration, the individual can participate in the collective without having to renounce his or her own interests. But in reality, the situation is often more complex. Individuals are obliged to suppress their inner selves and ignore their intuitions and desires. They sell their labor power, and are expected, in return, not to disrupt the balance of the system they serve.

The human struggle consists of trying to remain true to oneself while taking part in a society that has other objectives. For many, the resolution of this conflict leads to a genuine sense of fulfillment, for society offers many benefits that a lone individual could never access. Still, the persistence of diseases of civilization testifies to the fact that this resolution has never been an easy one, and, for some, the cost of submission and self-suppression has been intolerably high. If these diseases are particularly prevalent today, it is because individual intuitions and societal norms are more divergent than ever before. The ancient ideal of a harmonious balance between personal and societal equilibrium is hopelessly out of step with the times.

We have lost our intuitive equilibrium, defined by Aristotle as the pursuit of a happy medium, which his contemplation of nature, his understanding of the function of humors in the human body, and his meditations on the stability of societies all led him to embrace. This equilibrium was an *end in itself*, since harmony was to be sought for its own sake, as a thing of beauty and a source of joy.

But in our time, equilibrium has become a means to an end.[25] It is no longer a personal, artistic, or philosophical objective, but rather, a

[25] It is possible to date this change back to 1942. During the war, the nascent field of cybernetics introduced a new model of equilibrium, inspired not by nature, but by machines, and more specifically, by the anti-aircraft missile launchers that the American government had asked Norbert Wiener to develop. Wiener understood that when it came to launching a missile, balance was simply a means to an end. The goal was to hit the target. And it was with respect to this goal that the missile's trajectory had to be adjusted, a little farther to the left or right. Another classic example is that of the thermostat. The aim is to keep the temperature of a room at 66° F, and the operation of

process that allows us to conform to an extrinsically determined norm. Indeed, the goal of a course of action is typically defined from the outside, dictated, for example, by the imperatives of performance, profitability, or cost reduction. Normative equilibrium, which can dispense altogether with the happy medium when it is interpreted in terms of technological constraints, has at this point displaced the notion of intuitive equilibrium. The disjunction between the two has taken root, and only becomes more entrenched as an endless succession of new norms are issued, some of them having no correspondence whatsoever to lived experience. Intuition, the internal compass that once allowed each of us to distinguish between too much and too little, no longer has a voice.

To illustrate this transition from equilibrium as an end in itself to equilibrium as a means, no analogy is more instructive than a comparison of two types of weighing scales: old-fashioned twin-pan balance scales and modern electronic scales. The former, which corresponds to the Aristotelian concept of balance, allows us to visualize the happy medium. We see which side the scale is leaning toward, and thus, intuitively, we can discern what constitutes too much or too little. This technical object, now a universal symbol, has nonetheless been displaced by the electronic scale. And what does it show us? A number. Where balance is concerned, the intuitive dimension, foundational though it may have been, has long since been forgotten.

It must be rediscovered. For the individual, this goal is not unattainable. Reconnecting with our intuition, listening to our bodies, sleeping when we need to, and above all, looking within ourselves for other adventurous and inspiring imbalances, may be the start of a transformation. After all, isn't the soul the fundamental imbalance that animates each of us? Often, it is merely waiting to be reawakened! To consciously nurture one's own imbalances, to reshape body and soul so

the heater is regulated as a function of this target temperature. Wiener and other proponents of cybernetics used the same principles to explain that the biochemical regulation of the human body was typically just a means to maintain homeostasis, a model that definitively dispensed with the Aristotelian conception of the humors.

that they can transcend their limitations, this is the other, higher goal that gives meaning to the mastery of balance. This is precisely what the dancer does, when her movements take flight, and her gestures move beyond the sphere of everyday actions, to express an uncontainable power, liberated from the constraints of gravity. Suddenly suspended, the difficulty of living is replaced by pure freedom, transfigured by a corporeal exhilaration that radiates vitality through the arms, hands, and face.

Here, again, is the fire—the other fire—no longer that of burnout, but the flame that symbolizes the vibration of life in its purest form, as expressed by Paul Valéry in *L'Âme et la Danse* (published in English as *Dance and the Soul*), where he compares the dancer to a salamander in the fire: "this supremacy of tension, and this whirling into the greatest agility humanly possible, have the virtues and the powers of flame."[26] The meaning of everything is suddenly altered; the fire that once threatened to destroy has become a source of liberation and transformation. And this is only the beginning.

Still, on a societal level, the call to reconnect with our intuition is not enough. Certainly, the intolerable sensations and perceptions that afflict us constitute a call for changes to our systems of production and consumption, but how can we ensure that this call will be heard? The dominant systems appear stronger than ever, and theirs is a violence that muffles all other sounds. This is why it seems that the time has come for a new pact. The political philosophers of the eighteenth century developed the notion of a social contract to counteract the instability inherent in a "state of nature" which they envisioned as war of all against all—what we now call deregulation. Thus, they proposed a natural contract. To assure mankind's continued survival, they saw the need for an agreement by which all individuals would renounce their claim to the use of excessive force.

Three centuries later, we are in need of a new pact: not a natural contract this time, but a technological one, to act as a firewall, and to

26 Paul Valéry (trans. Dorothy Bussy), *Dance and the Soul*. London, J. Lehmann, 1951, p. 77.

affirm that our primary objective is the preservation of the human race and the biosphere that sustains us. Our systems of development must therefore work in the service of this goal, renouncing the violent methods they once employed. This philosophical notion is not a simple concept. In its modern form, it has already resulted in laws that helped to establish the relatively peaceful conditions we currently enjoy. In its postmodern form—that of a technological contract—it could, in the future, serve as a regulative ideal, to reign in our excesses before they cause us harm, and to ensure that all of us may experience the kind of idleness that is essential to all art, all philosophy and all contemplation.

Part IV

Postface to the English Edition

Burnout and energy

I must begin this postface by offering my sincere thanks to Patricia Pisters and Bernd Herzogenrath for making this book available to English-speaking audiences, and for giving me the opportunity, in the pages that follow, to further reflect on some of the topics examined in the French edition of *Global Burnout*. An important observation that emerges from this exploration of burnout is that the exhaustion experienced by those who sacrifice too much of themselves to the system they serve occurs within the larger context of a civilization which is itself burning through its resources, its fuel and, ultimately the entire biosphere. We have described burnout as a "mirror disorder," to signify that the suffering inflicted on individual members of society mirrors the abuse being perpetrated upon the planet. The system and its sub-systems display analogous patterns of behaviour and seem to be capable of cross-contamination through mutual imitation. But, how is this possible? What is the relationship between the phenomena we have observed? These are the questions we will attempt to analyse in the pages that follow.

Accounts of exhaustion and fatigue, questions about the relationship between individual and social factors contributing to burnout, and promises of a new "pact with technology" all seem to touch upon a collective blind spot, a kind of "dark zone"—to use an expression favoured by Simondon—which we will now attempt to infuse with light. What these different dimensions of the burnout question have in common is a connection to what we commonly refer to as *energy*. Energy deficits, fatigue, and even the frenetic surpluses of energy that are the counterpart to exhaustion; concerns about the energetic expenditures of large businesses, or *a fortiori*, of megacities that flood the night sky with light at a time when excessive reliance on fossil fuels is already choking the biosphere, this is the stage on which the phenomenon of *global burnout* is playing out. But what are the energies in question? Where do they come from, and how are they depleted? What is the connection between the energy exerted by a worker struggling to complete a task, the nuclear energy that in many countries still provides electricity to power computer screens and microprocessors, and that other, primal energy that makes life possible? Moreover, is there something that cuts across all of these dimensions, some essence that we can extract through philosophical analysis? Starting from this multiplicity of concrete examples, we will try to work our way back to the abstract concept of that strange "reality" we call energy.

The narrow perspective, which we categorically reject, would assert that there is, in fact, *no* connection between the organization of our work environment and the exhaustion of environmental resources. This argument rests upon the principle of compartmentalization. The burnout suffered by an individual is the result of a personal trajectory that leads her to reject a work situation she cannot abide, because it is toxic or hostile to her values. Why should we suppose that a link could be established between this professional problem and a civilization whose every desire is satisfied by access to oil, gas and electricity? *A priori*, there is none. But wouldn't it be interesting to construct one? Connections do not pre-exist insight; they are, rather, its products, which must be judged on the basis of their pertinence. Now, in this case, it seems clear that if we do not ordinarily draw connections between these phenomena, it is because the dualism that separates mind from matter constitutes a deeply ingrained intellectual framework, locking us into certain ways of thinking and preventing us from establishing certain relationships. We assume that individual problems linked to the organization of the work environment are purely an issue for social psychology, or more broadly, for social sciences concerned with the human mind. At the opposite extreme, techno-scientific aspects of energy, notably including the sources of fuel that power our machines, are firmly situated within the material sphere. Between these two realms there is little contact, let alone connection: the case seems to be settled.

Yet, if we dare to break down two of the principal barriers that stand in our path, we can shed new light on the situation. First of all, we must overcome the prohibitions that discourage us from contemplating energy, recognizing it, instead, as one of the keys to understanding our civilization. In so doing, we become aware that the domains of mind and matter, ordinarily kept separate, in fact share a common feature: both are arenas of energetic exchange. The second intellectual barrier to overcome is the conviction that certain kinds of energy are real, while others are purely metaphorical. According to this perspective, it is acceptable to speak of oil-based energy, whereas it is a misuse of language to refer to the energy of a person engaged in work. But, if we disregard this prohibition and resolve to consider the different types of energy in a democratic manner, putting them all on equal footing, we begin to notice certain similarities that enrich our reflections: in both of these cases, there is energy at stake, in both cases, some kind of "work" is performed, and in both cases, the energy involved is in limited supply and can be depleted. Within this philosophically open-minded experimental framework, we are able to construct an analogy.

We test the validity of this analogy ourselves every time we travel to a new location. Cities have different energetic patterns, each as distinctive as a signature. The energy of New York, rhythmic, fast-paced, decisive, and free, exerts its pull on pedestrians, speeding the cadence of their feet and their thoughts. Seoul, more frenetic, hyperactive, consumption-driven one moment, and playful the next, leaves its imprint on people, or more precisely, transmits to them an energy that captures the spirit of the city—the word "imprint" suggests something too static. The contagion that spreads between people and places constitutes an anthropologically significant fact. It is as if the patterns of energetic expenditure displayed by visitors to a place were a function of the number of people they encounter, the frequency of their voices, the signals from their electronic devices, the noise from their engines, and the endless interactions between them. Human beings adapt quickly to these environmental cues. It would be impossible, standing on the *Terrazza dell'infinito* in Ravello, to remain under the sway of electronic rhythms. The energy of the place imposes serenity and detachment. Inversely, it becomes difficult to maintain a carefree attitude in a subway station where the faces of fellow commuters, marked by the cares of the workaday world, display a sort of listless neutrality. The influence of the collective partly accounts for this kind of contagion. The phenomenon of mimesis certainly plays a role. But something else is also happening: there is real communication that occurs, in these zones of coincidence, between a place and the people who pass through it. Human beings are very sensitive to energy—malleable, even. Filmmakers, photographers, writers, and choreographers are aware of this: patterns of energy are palpable, and deserve to be acknowledged as such by the field of philosophy. The energy in question need not be frenetic, or technical. In *The Magic Mountain*, Thomas Mann shows how the sickly, tepid energy of a sanatorium strips Hans Castorp's soul of its vitality, acting upon his spirit like a black hole that sucks in the intentions of a healthy mind and distils them into a miasma of fatigue and oblivion. This is a novel animated by the energies of neurasthenia. How could anyone think to reduce it to a simple psychological investigation, when it presents an evocation of a place, an institution, a relationship with nature, and ultimately, a conception of European culture? Artists seek to capture the energies that occupy the space between mind and matter. Why, then, should philosophers be determined to do without them?

We must attempt a phenomenological description of human energy, for it is this energy, and its depletion, that are at stake in the case of burnout. We must also ask ourselves why the phenomenological tradition has, for so long, been reluctant to consider energy as a real phenomenon. We lean habitually on notions of mind and body, as if they were passive substances. But we must observe them *in action*, or to use the Aristotelian term, in their *energeia*. Approaching them from this perspective, the first reality we encounter is the musculature of the body. Its characteristics include robustness, solidity, and vigour. By assessing its physical strength and tone, weighted against the variables of age and gender, we can determine our subject's health, vivacity, constitution, and resistance. In the motion of the muscles, we can also detect calmness and tranquillity, languor, fatigue, weariness or stress, which is energy turned taut and aggressive. Vocal modulation, facial expression, eye contact, hand gestures, movement of the neck, everything that classical rhetoric calls *actio* expresses these bodily manifestations of energy. The body is a direct extension of the mind. Philosophy has wedded itself to a false dichotomy by insisting on the separation of mind and body. By decrypting the non-verbal language of the body, we can, to an extent, extrapolate intellectual and moral characteristics based on physical cues. Firmness, obstinacy, resilience, equilibrium, fragility, dynamism, serenity, docility, apathy: these core personality traits are encoded in our physical postures, sensed rather than expressed, subliminally detected rather than consciously articulated. Our relationships are shaped by these perceptions, which determine our attractions and repulsions, our sympathies and our affections.

Returning now to our guiding question, what connections can we establish between these human energies and the energy that fuels our civilization? For, a connection does exist. To refuse to recognize it, we would have to subscribe to an eternal account of anthropology, in which our heroes, human beings, remained forever self-contained and unchangeable. Their material, technological and *energetic* environment would have little more than a superficial effect on them. They would change the planet, contemplate ideas and construct extraordinary cities; they would exploit all available resources and even go so far as to modify the climate, albeit involuntarily. But they themselves would not change, or only very slightly. They would remain the one constant unaffected by time, spectators to history. It is impossible, of course, to believe in this poetic narrative. Our habits, our computers, even our modes of transport modify us. And all of this infrastructure depends on the enormous quantities of energy that human beings capture and harness. We are what we do. But how should we interpret this declaration today? Is its modern equivalent *we are the energy that we consume*?

The invisibility of energy

The flora of the Jurassic Era, which withered and died over the course of an unimaginable autumn, are separated from us by one hundred and fifty million years. At that time, luxurious jungles, giant ferns, and Ginkgo trees covered the earth, providing shelter for the earliest birds. Alongside them were dinosaurs—herbivorous Sauropods, Diplodocus and Brachiosaurus, and the predators that hunted them, drawn to their blood and their flesh. There were also generation upon generation of marine crocodiles and other peculiar animals that flourished for millions of years in this sunny, oxygen-rich environment, then decomposed at length. Some of their remains wound up covered in sediment, sometimes at the bottom of the sea, mixing with plankton, algae, and alluvia, a substrate of once-living matter, soon to be flattened by layers of silt and sand, buried beneath mineral shale, and trapped under molten, metamorphic rock. Over time, this decomposing matter would form kerogen, an insoluble organic substance that accumulates in mineral deposits. Chemists explain that over millions of years, this kerogen, preserved in reservoirs pushed deeper and deeper below the earth's surface, was subjected to extremely high temperatures and pressure, forcing out oxygen and water and resulting in an increased concentration of hydrocarbons. "Oil! Oil!" would come the cry, much later on.

Philosophy is born out of wonder, just as oil is born of organic matter. In each case, a long period of metamorphosis, followed by painstaking refinement, is required in order to produce a usable substance. But without wonder, there is no philosophy, just as without life there would be no oil. And what is there to inspire our wonder, if not the curious link between the organic waste products of the Jurassic Era and the world we know today. The one holds the *possibility* of the other. For what is today a routine occurrence—a cross-country drive behind the wheel of a car weighing nearly a tonne and a half, that two adult humans would struggle to push for even twenty meters—would be impossible without this dark substance, which offers, to those who know how to transform it, the power to desire things that no human being previously would have dared to wish for. *Energy is the possibility of desire.* If our civilization is so full of desires, so insatiable in its appetites, inventive in its fantasies and impatient for their gratification, it is because we have access to this potion for which the epithet "magic" is wholly inadequate. The objectives we have set for ourselves—for example, lifting a forty-tonne aeroplane miles off the ground in order to transport eight hundred people to the opposite hemisphere—would be unthinkable but for the existence of a fuel that can be converted into a force both colossally powerful and finely manipulable. Without it, dreams of air travel would have never have progressed beyond the sketches in Leonardo's notebooks.

The wonder that we are trying now to cultivate is elicited not only by the improbability of this encounter between Jurassic vegetation and the sometimes capricious fancies of highly evolved human beings, but also by the fact that this energy goes virtually unnoticed. It has become banal. We think it only normal that we should be able to pump out petrol at will, and we grumble when the prices increase . . . The banality of miracles is a strangely charming feature of an outlook grounded in common sense; whatever is familiar fails to thrill us—we grow inured to wonders, blasé about innovation. This also happens to be the feature that most clearly distinguishes common sense from philosophy or art. The former is awed by things that diverge completely from everyday experience, by whatever is new, bizarre, extraordinary. Only the most improbable event sets its cognitive wheels spinning; like a spider perched on its web, it is roused to action only when it senses something new in its environment. In contrast, art, poetry, and even philosophy—which often draws from the same sources of inspiration—tend to disregard oddities in favour of the familiar, whose intimate mysteries they seek to uncover. Reality, for those who see it clearly, is stranger than the sensationalized stories that draw attention. It is the banal that dizzies us with its depth. It is the ordinary that sparks our curiosity and keeps us awake at night. So it is with oil, hundreds of thousands of barrels of which are bought and sold each day.

A single cup of this opaque liquid contains the same amount of energy that a manual labourer expends over four long months. We can calculate this because different forms of energy are convertible and can thus, in theory, be compared. It appears, then, that this labourer, whose solid, well-trained muscles work steadily for eight hours a day, engaged in what feels to him like back-breaking work, ultimately exerts an amount of force that could be comfortably contained within a small flask. Aladdin's lamp was by no means a greater marvel, apart from the fact that it was treated as one. We, on the other hand, have all but ceased to notice the enchantment of this energy, to which we entrust our everyday miracles. What should be mind-boggling has become banal. Within the space of a few decades, human beings have classified as "normal" the fact that we have at our constant disposal a power far greater than our own. This illustrates the extent to which normality is relative, and how, like comfort, it seems in certain parts of the world to be entirely taken for granted. The power contained within our energy sources is as improbable as our habituation to the wonders they hold.

The figure of Nikola Tesla presents another perspective on the fascinating aspects of this energy which have nonetheless receded to the edges of our consciousness. His work belongs to the heroic period that saw the electrification of America, funded by the likes of J.P. Morgan, John D. Rockefeller and George Westinghouse. Aerial cables were being strung through America's cities, while the pioneers of the distribution networks vied for control over their organization. Among them, Tesla, a Serbian-American inventor, visionary and eccentric known as the "electrical wizard," who filed more than three hundred patents for his inventions, which included the radar, the neon tube, the transformer and the remote control. He also had the prescience to predict that, one day, electromagnetic waves would carry human voices around the world.

The task at hand, however, was to render electrical energy *visible*, to make a spectacle of this new source of power poised to dethrone human, animal, mechanical, wind and hydraulic energy sources. The city chronicles of the era attest to the public's appetite for high-voltage performances, set against a backdrop of copper wires. So it was that Tesla, solitary and moody by nature, turned showman in order to showcase his passion. At private dinners or on stage, he provided demonstrations of intensity, frequency and short-circuits, producing arcs of electricity, bolts of lightning and balls of fire. "His showmanship," writes Jean Echenoz, who paints a magnificent portrait of this electrical wizard and his enchanting displays, "wins over crowds flabbergasted by his performances and his variety of props."[1] A series of demonstrations was thus organized around these new energies. They came to a crescendo with the "War of Currents," a technological and economic battle that pitted Edison, proponent of the direct current, against Tesla, inventor of the alternating current. Edison's goal was to prove that his adversary's creations were mortally dangerous. To bolster his case, he electrocuted chickens, sheep and cattle, all before an audience, in the middle of New York City. To drive home the point, he did the same to an elephant that had recently killed three circus employees. Shot through with thousands of volts of electricity, the pachyderm flopped to the ground as a crowd of spectators looked on, entranced. Continuing his campaign of defamation, he designed the first electric chair, thus inventing a new means of killing. Here was energy revealed in all its power; no more could anyone doubt that it had the capacity to change lives . . .

Edison did not triumph in the end, however, because alternating current can travel across longer distances than direct current, on account of its higher voltage. Soon, networks were put in place, power plants were built far outside the city limits, and almost everyone forgot the spectacular demonstrations put on by these pioneers. But what endures from this brief moment in history is the desire to make energy *visible*, and in so doing, to gain awareness of its potential. Perhaps, to our jaded eyes, there is a childish quality to these spectacles. We who

1 J. Echenoz (trans. Linda Coverdale), *Lightning* (*Des éclairs*), New York, The New Press, 2011; see also J. O'Neill, *Prodigal Genius: The Life of Nikola Tesla*, New York, Cosimo, Inc., 2006. In Brazil, the *Instituto Tesla* pursues research inspired by the Serbo-American inventor's vision of "free energy."

have "matured," whose relationship with the magic of electricity is now either utilitarian, via the power switch, or commercial, via our monthly bills, would not be so easily awed by these simple demonstrations. Familiarity has gotten the better of wonder. And yet, on reflection, what has really changed, apart from the habituation that keeps us from noticing energy?

Often, it is true, every effort is made to obscure from our view the sources of the energy we consume. The nuclear power industry is a prime example of this. In a probing essay devoted to this topic, Jean-Jacques Delfour shares the following analysis: "Nuclear power is everywhere; its effects on us are felt constantly, and yet, almost nowhere is it actually visible—it eludes our grasp. This paradoxical duality is a fact: a massive, permanent reality that has spread to every corner of the globe, while remaining cloaked in secrecy, quasi-absent, confidential, taboo."[2] The physical reactions that take place inside a nuclear power plant are hidden from view. A handful of diagrams and a few scant images, always the same, might provide some information, but the necessity of confinement renders them distant and inaccessible. This invisibility of nuclear energy is further reinforced when we consider radioactivity. It is intangible, odourless, unobservable: just the movement of a needle on a dial, or a sequence of numbers. It is this quality of being imperceptible yet mortally dangerous that caused such unease at the time of the Fukushima disaster. The contamination of the air, soil, water, flora and fauna is certain, but undetectable to our senses. For human beings, seeing is believing. But here, everything is hidden, concealed from everyone except a few scientists with a kind of monopoly on knowledge. Even the victims of the accident are kept at a distance from the cameras. Cancers triggered by radiation exposure may not appear for many years, and are not always easily detected. "The multi-faceted invisibility of nuclear power"[3] has a wide variety of

[2] J.-J. Delfour, *La condition nucléaire. Réflexions sur la situation atomique de l'humanité*, Montreuil, Editions L'échappée, 2014, p. 12.

[3] *Ibid.*, p. 256.

causes, but all of them serve to keep it at a distance, far away from public scrutiny.

This context sheds new light on the debate over renewable energy. Unlike oil, that miracle made commonplace, unlike electricity, that magical force celebrated by Tesla but no longer a source of wonder to a populace spoiled by modern conveniences, unlike nuclear power, kept out of sight and out of mind, renewable energy unapologetically takes up space and catches the eye. What could be more visible than the enormous wind turbines invading the countryside, like modern descendants of the windmills that menaced Don Quixote in La Mancha? Here, the strategy is not at all one of retreat, but of conspicuous display. In northern Holland, these enormous propellers affixed to gigantic masts dominate the view, adding verticality and movement to an otherwise flat, horizontal landscape. The entire space appears transformed into a giant machine, and the impression of *work*—the literal translation of the Greek word *energeia*—radiates from this landscape, impossible to miss. In much the same way, solar energy flaunts its presence. On rooftops, in public spaces or in fields, these prominent panels display their dark reflective surfaces for all to see, as if to draw attention to their virtues. They counter the invisibility of nuclear energy with a conspicuousness that announces "We've got nothing to hide."

And it is precisely this conspicuousness that their detractors complain about. Solar panels turn buildings into eyesores, and wind farms are a blight on pastoral landscapes—these are two of the arguments frequently advanced. Here again, the debate centres around visibility. There is a strong desire to prohibit energy production from making itself conspicuous or from colonizing what remains of the "natural world," even as we allow it to play a decisive role in our daily lives. The famous slogan *Not in my backyard* expresses the ambiguity of a desire that we demand to see fulfilled while turning our backs on the means of its fulfillment.

What does this debate teach us, if not that our relationship with energy is troubled, noncommittal and often thoughtless? These games of hide and seek are a testament to our malaise. We want energy, but at the same time, we don't want it. . . What does this paradox signify? Of what malady is it the symptom, and how can we account for it? These are the kinds of questions that must guide us. Energy, in the broadest sense of the term, is one of the most deeply repressed elements in our way of thinking about the world. We must now attempt to understand the reasons for this. In fact, it is only through a better understanding of this repression and its causes that we can hope to restore energy to its rightful place, which is to say a central place, since it represents the possibility of desire. This applies not only to physical energy, but also to the psychic energy that allows us to live and to be, and which sometimes, when exhausted, brings both living and being to a grinding halt. In psychological as well as physical terms, energy is the possibility of desire.

The causes of repression

We consume energy with reckless abandon, but we almost never think about it. In Western traditions it has been pushed aside, as if it did not fit within our interpretive framework. Science and technology allow it to play a central role, but philosophy and culture alike ignore it, with a few important exceptions to which we will later return. This situation recalls the status of technology in the philosophical thought of the last century. At first neglected and considered unworthy of interest, later brought to the forefront, notably by Heidegger and Simondon, it has become an indispensable topic of reflection for understanding the way we live. Now, it is time for energy to come into its own. A major economic, geopolitical and technological force, it deserves to be taken seriously as a philosophical concern, for its effects extend even as far as our own psyches.

Ontological causes of repression

A number of factors help to account for our blind spot concerning energy. The first is ontological: our tradition is structured around the dualism of mind versus matter, which informs our conception of nature, the body, and life itself. Competing philosophical schools argued about whether mind or matter had primacy, giving rise to various forms of spiritualism and materialism. But few indeed were those who managed to see beyond this dualist framework, to insist upon the relevance of a third reality: energy.

It was only at the periphery of this mind–matter division that considerations of energy began to emerge, albeit lacking unity and rarely cutting across disciplines. Matter could not remain completely passive. Aristotle, the great Founding Father of philosophy, had the felicitous idea to attribute to matter either power (*dynamis*, the potential for action), or energy (*energeia*, power in action). The mind, likewise, could not simply exist, with no motivation or driving force: it was bestowed with enthusiasm, will, desire, or in times of trouble, fatigue, melancholy, even burnout. These energies are always circumstantial. Their effects are ancillary to the primary substances of mind and matter, although one might well wonder what would become of these substances without the energy that animates them.

It was the French philosopher Gilbert Simondon (1924–1989) who first had the insight to observe that, having establishing this notion of *energeia*, Aristotle nonetheless failed to give it its proper due in his analysis of the process of individuation. In Simondon's own famous analysis of the "physico-biological genesis of the individual,"[4] he notes that the two categories Aristotle calls upon to explain the formation of a particular reality are matter, ὑλο- (*hylo-*) and form, μορφή (*morphē*). The intersection of these two terms produces what he described as the hylomorphic schema, which is an explication of individuation according to which form is imposed on passive matter, in much the same way that a human form is imposed on clay to produce a statue of Pericles.

4 G. Simondon, *L'individu et sa genèse physico-biologique* [*The Physico-Biological Genesis of the Individual*], Grenoble, Million, 1988. See also P. Chabot, *The Philosophy of Simondon*, London, Bloomsbury, 2013, translated by Graeme Krikpatrick and Aliza Krefetz.

This hylomorphic explanation was of major importance, according to Simondon. Vestiges of it can still be seen in certain attitudes toward education, which postulate that a young child is a passive receptacle, like human modelling clay (the "matter") to be moulded with rules, which correspond to Aristotelian forms. In other domains, such as political science, which tends to conceive of the masses as a chaotic force upon which speech acts as an organizing principle, hylomorphism was like the first matrix of a constantly reiterated explanation. For every permutation of reality, Western thought sought to distinguish passive matter from its active form. But it unduly simplified the complexity of individuation by reducing it to this over-generalized schema, whose principal defect is that it completely neglects, and even excludes, the energetic dimension of the operation. For "it is as *forces* that matter and form are brought together,"[5] explains Simondon in his detailed analysis of the process of making a brick. Clay is not "passive matter": it has thermal and molecular energetic properties. And the mould that compresses the clay to make the brick itself also acts as an energetic force. Aristotle, however, neglected this element, and an entire tradition has followed in his footsteps, pushing energy back into the realm of hard to explain mysteries, favouring the almost Platonic clarity of a form that resembles an idea, and the questionable premise of a "passive matter," an entity that is nowhere to be found in nature.

The Aristotelean choice, to which history paid tribute by employing it for more than two thousand years, was one of expedience. It makes perfect sense if we consider that matter and form are simple and easy to use categories, useful for clarifying ideas and constructing analyses, whereas energy was still a messy and confusing reality for a Greek philosopher hundreds of years before the Common Era. Including it in the equation might have obliged him to sacrifice some of the clarity of the analysis, for language and energy accommodate each other poorly. To speak of energy is to invoke the inexplicable—which may not be what we expect of an explanation.

[5] G. Simondon, *ibid.*, p. 39.

Western philosophy has been held hostage to the dual categories of "spiritualism" and "materialism." Rare indeed are those who have attempted to formulate a theory of energeticism. Among these heretics was the Russian-German chemist Wilhelm Ostwald, Nobel Prize winner for chemistry in 1909, whose advocacy on behalf of energeticism influenced Nietzsche and his notion of the will to power, itself a form of energy.[6] The secondary ranking of energy is typically Western. Unlike traditional Eastern thought, which is more concerned with becoming than being, with the energy of metamorphosis rather than the stability of substance, with subtle fluids, breath and chakras, rather than the organs and their functions, European thought granted energy at most a secondary status, at the margins of its central categories. The important things were mind and matter, whose binary opposition constitutes the major nexus from which Western culture, and its collective unconscious, emanates.

Energy is thus the least acknowledged element within the Western philosophical tradition, whereas it is central to the Eastern understanding of the world and of humankind. Its repression may in fact constitute the biggest difference between Eastern and Western thought. It is explained by the particular philosophical groundwork set in place by Plato and, even more decisively, by Aristotle. Before them, philosophical inquiries into the nature of energy were indeed present, and even central. In the great philosophical poems composed by the Pre-Socratics, energy assumes a primary role. Heraclitus perceived an interplay of forces in perpetual flux, which led him to remark that "war is the father of all." Anaximander identified, at the centre of reality, an ἄπειρον (*apeiron*), a sort of indeterminate, undifferentiated substance, without shape or form, but pulsating with the energetic potentialities of the fully formed entities it would give rise to. Empedocles, likewise, assigned a central role to the energetic exchanges between particles, in

6 See D. Ghesquier-Pourcin, *Ostwald et le monisme*, in D. Ghesquier-Pourcin, M. Guedj, G. Gohau and M. Party, *Energie, science et philosophie. Les formes de l'énergétisme et leur influence sur la pensée*, Paris, Hermann, 2010, p. 83.

what was to be the earliest precursor to atomic physics. Anaxagoras, for his part, suggested that all things proceeded from the νοῦς (*noùs*), a principle that is, in essence, a major, universal force of energy. These philosophers, who hailed from Ionia, on the coast of modern-day Turkey, or from a few sun-scorched islands nearby, wrote well before the establishment of philosophy—or at least, its Athenian incarnation. In according a primary role to energy, they stayed close to the ancient myths and religions which still held sway. The ancient Egyptians, whose religion had a well-documented influence on Greek thought, dedicated their most fervent worship to the sun god Ra. From a northerly vantage point, it can be difficult to fathom the extent of this veneration for the sun, but the further south one goes, whether physically or in the mind's eye, the more the abundant power of the universe's biggest nuclear plant leaves its mark on the flora and fauna, as well as the skin, the habits and the minds of those it touches. In making the Sun the analogue of Goodness, thus placing it at the summit of the world of ideas that served as his philosophical pantheon, Plato, too, affirms his allegiance to this tradition of people who cannot bear the darkness of the caves, where slaves of illusion languish in the shadows, seeking instead to move forward, unbound, into the reality of light. The statement that most meaningfully captures the sun-centric Platonic outlook is surely this: "We can easily forgive a child who is afraid of the dark; the real tragedy of life is when men are afraid of the light."

But Plato is more than a child of the Sun. He is also a wise crafter of language, a cunning master of dialectics who seeks, by defining things with precision and giving priority to what he calls the "the rectitude of their denominations," to systematically record all that is real and organize it into categories. Aristotle, even more so than Plato, would formalize this powerful imposition of the order of language onto the chaotic and inchoate world of sensory experience; with all the force of his formidable, methodical mind, he would marshal the singularities of individual phenomena into a regimented framework of genera, species and specific differences, organized according to a rigorous logic. This is how science was born, through the imposition of linguistic order onto a range of sensations which had hitherto known no organizing principles beyond the general schemas of perception and action. The movement from these habitual schemas, typical of *Homo faber*, to categories of understanding, constitutes one of the major dimensions early Western philosophy.

And yet, an essential element underpinning this philosophy was a wilful disregard for energy. To put it another way, the establishment of this philosophical foundation was only made possible by minimizing the role of energy to the maximum extent. Philosophical order was established by sweeping energy to the side, and treating it as the "other." This was a decisive action, an intellectual gesture whose consequences are still felt today. We must trace its development, if we are to understand our power-based civilization and the hold it has on our psyches—inspiring us or exhausting us to the point of burnout—and if we are to find a way to curtail its violence. The gesture that separates energy from language is integral to Western thought—and not Eastern thought, it must be emphasized—because it assumes that energy and language belong to two different orders, and correspond to two perspectives on reality that are incompatible, or at least, that cannot be accessed simultaneously. This does not mean that no relationship can exist between energy and language; such relationships are numerous, culminating in a modern world where power and information are inextricably linked. But this contemporary link does not change the fact that a real gulf exists between the two dimensions of experience that energy and language represent. Energetic dynamism and linguistic analyticism constitute two opposite poles whose problematic relationship has shaped the Western world.

Cultural causes of repression

It must be acknowledged—and here we hit upon a cultural reason for its repression—that energy belongs to that order of elusive realities that defy our intelligence and seem to constitute the other side of reason, its dark, hidden face. Bergson noted that our intelligence is adapted for contemplating stable, solid, fixed realities, like stones and tables. This observation affirms how ill-suited it is for grasping energy's potential, and indeed, its near-magical power, to endlessly transform all that exists.

Western culture has, moreover, harshly stigmatized those intellectuals who sought to *contemplate* this elusive reality. To "contemplate" it, which means not just citing physics equations and leaving scientists the task of explaining its behaviour, but to construct a concept of energy using language as the building material. This desire to express the reality and the importance of energy was motivated by the will to show that energy was also a human reality. It was not just a force emitted by atoms, black holes, the sun or burning oil, but a concept that could help us to describe psychological behaviours, desires, or, even more elusive, perceptions, as when a person or place is said to radiate a particular type of energy. Judgements of this kind have often been denounced. Anyone who talks about energy in a way that goes beyond scientific usage is at risk of being dismissed or ridiculed. We have only to look at the sarcastic responses that greeted Bergson's *Spiritual Energy*,[7] Jung's *On Psychic Energy*[8] or Teilhard de Chardin's *Human Energy*.[9] These transgressive thinkers, who dared to name that which others refused to even consider, of course had their disciples and admirers. But a majority of commentaries concerning them were frequently hostile. They were viewed as would-be mystics and visionaries and criticized for turning their attention to the "insensible perceptions" that had once been used as the basis for a philosophy of mind, or more broadly, a science of spiritual matters. Critics could not understand their audacity in taking a well-defined scientific term and applying it to something as indefinite and contradictory as the human mind.

The dominant culture's defence mechanism was to exclude energy, relegating it to the strange and sublime hodgepodge of counter-cultural

7 Bergson, H. *L'énergie spirituelle*, Paris, PUF, 1959 (1st edition 1919).

8 Jung, C.G. "On Psychic Energy" in *On the Nature of the Psyche*, Princeton, Princeton University Press, 1960.

9 Teilhard de Chardin, P. *L'énergie humaine*, Paris, Seuil, 1962.

sub-groups that included illuminism, alchemy, esotericism, magnetism, parapsychology, New-Age psychology, yoga and an assortment of other practices, whose proponents were inevitably suspected—sometimes rightly so—of abusing illegal substances and filling their own minds with pipe dreams. Physicists, chemists, geologists and stock market speculators can talk about energy as much as they want. But a philosopher or psychologist who so much as mentions the word is suspected of having spent too much time in the deserts around Los Angeles, in Pondicherry or perhaps Guatemala, following in the footsteps of Castaneda. They are called, among other things, *travellers*, a label which emphasizes that these energies are "foreign" to us.

Energy enthusiasts are subjected to a sort of trial by metaphor. Accusing them of deviance, their prosecutors start from the assumption that there exists one "genuine" variety of energy, plus an assortment of other "*je-ne-sais-quoi*"s described as "energies" only for the sake of analogy or convenience. The relationship between the primary signification and these secondary metaphors parallels the relationship between any genuine article and a set of counterfeit knock-offs, with the same implication of false pretence and inauthenticity. This comparison supports the view that there is only one authentic form of energy—that which physics defines as the property of a system capable of producing a quantifiable amount of work—and that the other properties that are described, for lack of a better term, as psychic energy, creative energy, or sexual energy, are really only *pseudo*-energies. There is something paternalistic in this attitude, as if the agreement to refer to these newcomers as energies were merely a placating goodwill gesture. A preferable alternative, which we will adopt in the reflections that follow, would be a *familial* attitude, with a nod to Wittgenstein's notion of family resemblance, or better yet, an *amicable* attitude, meaning that every use of the term has its own *raison d'être* and that none will be given hierarchical priority over others. The high-energy physics conducted by CERN and the high-energy antics of the Roman eccentrics who populate Paolo Sorrentino's *La Grande Bellezza*, coexist as part of the multi-coloured tapestry of our modern world. There is no reason to valorize certain types of energy while denigrating others, on the pretext that relativism is to be avoided at all costs. These concepts belong to a shared network of significations, even as they very obviously refer to different things.

Adopting this attitude by no means obliges us to abandon definitions altogether. On the contrary, to borrow an expression from Paul Valéry, a "clean-up of the verbal situation"[10] is an indispensable step towards understanding this complex reality. But in acknowledging the multiplicity of meanings contained within this term, we leave behind the constraints of a narrow-minded scientism. If we examine the notion of energy as it pertains to physics, and then again in technological, philosophical and cultural contexts, the view that emerges is a surprising one. The concept, which starts off in the realm of the objective and experimental, soon reveals its geopolitical, financial, psychological and parapsychological nuances. They form a strange mosaic that cannot possibly be made to fit within a single category. The typical strategy, when confronted with such a fragmented concept, would be to examine the debris, matching each fragment *ad hoc* to the appropriate discipline: physics, technology, politics, ecology, every piece correctly categorized, with communication between categories only as circumstances warrant. But while each of these individual disciplines already provide us with a wealth of information—more than we could possibly hope to tally—there is a case to be made for a cross-discipline analysis that would attempt to establish relationships between these different approaches. The notion must remain fractured, fragmented, and for the most part "deterritorialized" as Deleuze, who was himself not exactly lacking in creative energy, would have it. The goal is not to come up with an unambiguous, all-purpose definition, nor to unearth some impossibly unifying kernel of wisdom, but to look within this multi-faceted reality for echoes, resonances, familial relationships, meeting points, and moments of insight that might shed some light on our problem. *Because,*

10 Translator's note: "nettoyage de la situation verbale"; this is a famous line from Valéry's essay on "Poésie et pensée abstraite (Poetry and abstract thought)."

now more than ever, energy has become our problem, on account of its dwindling availability, but also due to the fact that the insistence on constant, frenetic energization could prove lethal for certain people who feel their lives are devoted to a system that sucks up all of their energy. The theories we cling to, our habits, our fictions, our programs of action research all attest to the fact that this fuel source plays a crucial role in our relationship with a technocapitalist system and in the evolution of our mindset. We cannot afford to exclude certain fields of exploration *a priori*, on the grounds that they lack scientific rigour, or conversely, that they are excessively technical, nor can we afford to valorize some to the detriment of others. Philosophy is an ever-unfinished effort to organize a chaos which it plays a considerable role in creating. It is a means of establishing relationships, of finding passages, pathways and channels that cut through the infinite complexities of culture, bringing together disparate disciplines in the hopes of generating fresh insights. Its biggest enemy is the isolationist tendency to retreat into close-minded certainties. The closing of borders leads to ideological stagnation, narrow-mindedness, and the diffusion of stereotypes. If a philosophy of energy is to exist, it must remain fragmentary and open ended.

Social cause(s) of repression

In addition to these ontological and cultural causes, there is an important social factor that also helps to explain why energy is so seldom a topic of discussion or contemplation. To understand this factor, we would do well to take a step back and examine the situation of ancient civilizations. Who, within the social hierarchy, was tasked with the production of energy? The answer is simple. Energy was primarily generated by the bodies of slaves, who were perceived as soulless tools, or *instrumentum vocale*, as the Code of Justinian expressed it. They built roads, tilled the earth, manned the oars in the galleys of ships, and kept the millwheels turning. They were the energy converters of their time. Their daily ration of food was calibrated to keep their bodies burning as many joules of energy as their muscles were capable of expending, from morning to night. To fully understand the conquests of Rome, we must remember its insatiable thirst for energy, its need for a means to realize its lofty desires. The prisoners of war that the legions brought back in chains from Dacia, Egypt or Gaul were, in effect, human engines. The Greeks and the Persians did the same. The powerful in those days were almost invariably slaveholders, because the primary source of power was human labour. Yet few seemed to notice it. An entire geopolitical landscape was shaped by the quest for more bodies capable of labour; entire economic sectors depended on the purchase of men, women, and children, bought and resold as long as they were fit enough, still capable of work. But these slaves, who every day converted the gruel they were fed into muscular exertion, remained almost invisible: those who benefited from their efforts could scarcely be bothered to look and see who it was that carried their litters or turned the millwheels. Only every now and then would a poet stop to contemplate what others forgot to see, like Apuleius, in his *Metamorphoses*, where he describes the operation of a mill:

> I became totally absorbed in studying . . . the routine of this unpleasant establishment. As to the human contingent—what a crew!—their whole bodies picked out with livid weals, their whip-scarred backs shaded rather than covered by their tattered rags . . . There were branded foreheads . . . and fettered ankles; their faces were sallow, their eyes so bleared by the smoky heat of the furnaces that they were half blind.[11]

[11] Apuleius, *The Golden Ass, or Metamorphoses*, trans. E.J. Kenney, London, Penguin Books, 2004, Book IX, pp. 130–131; also cited by J.C. Debeir, J.P. Deléage and D. Hémery, in *Une Histoire de L'énergie*, Paris, Flammarion, 2013, p. 85. In their brilliant study of the history of energy, Debeir, Deléage and Hémery speculate that the abundant supply of human energy was one of the reasons the ancient Romans made little effort to exploit other sources of energy. "As far as mechanical energy is concerned," they write, "for as long as there prevailed a kind of growth based on the expansion of the servile labour force, and as long as they could draw upon a steady stream of prisoners of war to maintain the supply, as was the case in the second and first centuries B.C., not a single new energy-saving machine was widely adopted."

A similar description could be applied to many of the labourers who toiled through the Middle Ages, and even into Modern Times, when human beings continued to be used as human engines. Even if they weren't technically slaves, but serfs or members of the underclass, their lives were often equally arduous. Hauling boats along rivers, turning presses, pulling plows: there are countless examples of this human energy, exchanged for a bit of food or a meagre wage, that kept society running in the days before diesel engines.

The vestiges of this servile relationship continue to inform our mentality concerning energy. The slaves still go unnoticed; the entire system would be thrown off course if they were to call attention to themselves. To look too closely at the origins of movement or power is to occupy oneself unduly with unimportant minutia. The citizens of Athens liked to watch the triremes sailing off to sea, but barely gave a thought to the 170 oarsmen, sometimes free men, sometimes slaves, but always poor, whose exertions allowed the vessel to attain a speed of five knots. What went on in the galley was purely a technical question. As has been repeatedly shown, the foundations of Western philosophy were established against the backdrop of an aristocratism incapable of imagining the complex systems of power management that held it in place. A machine may also fill the role of the slave, who is unceremoniously discarded at the least sign of failure to perform. Gilbert Simondon was the first to make this comparison. The opening paragraph of his *Mode d'existence des objets techniques* concludes with this statement of intention: "An awareness of the modes of existence of technical objects must be brought about by philosophical thought, which finds itself with a duty to fulfill in this process analogous to the role it played in the abolition of slavery and the affirmation of human rights."[12] The same applies to the question of power, and from this perspective, the philosophy of energy is a continuation of the philosophy of technology.

[12] G. Simondon, *Du mode d'existence des objets techniques* [*On the Mode of Existence of Technical Objects*], Paris, Aubier, 1958 (ed. 1989, p. 9).

Slavery, is, fortunately, a distant reality for Western society today, but the slaveholder's mentality persists here and there, forming little islands of predatory thoughtlessness. If the question of energy is notably absent from our culture, it is because the availability of energy is seen as the normal state of affairs, when in actuality, it is something almost miraculous and difficult to procure. While driving through the countryside, we are more apt to turn our minds to thoughts of the appointment we are headed to, than to ponder the political and scientific ramifications of the labour that results from the combustion of oil in our fuel tank. For all we know, that oil might have come from Iraq, in which case it may have motivated a bomb attack, or Siberia, in which case it might be implicated in the repression of political activists. Then again, perhaps it came from Norway, Nigeria, or Venezuela. Even if we wanted to know, it would take extensive investigation to track down its provenance. In an earlier time, slaves had no names. Today, our petrol has no country of origin.

In his *Oil Notes*, geologist Rick Bass reflects on his work and on his mission as an oil hunter: to find black gold beneath American soil. His observations touch upon the Jurassic origins of oil deposits, his intuitions, the way he interprets the contours of a landscape, the possible presence of an underground reservoir of oil. He explains his distaste for "dirty" carbon and the pleasure he derives from "just go(ing) out and ... sink(ing) a hole in the ground, shov(ing) the pipe down there deep enough, until oil begins to flow up out of it, bubbling, with its rich smell of hiddenness and with the energy of discovery."[13] Over the course of his narrative, a gulf emerges between his research on the one hand, made more and more difficult due to dwindling oil reserves, and on the other hand, a human population unconcerned with the intricacies of oil refinement, blithely burning through millions of barrels of this unrenewable liquid resource each day. These two worlds are inextricably linked, yet entirely oblivious to one another. Bass hunts for oil while despising the oil companies whose interests he serves. And these

[13] R. Bass, *Oil Notes*, Lincoln, University of Nebraska Press, 2012, p. 1.

companies, for their part, remain unaware of and indifferent to his contempt. The ancient conflict between the patricians and their invisible slaves crops up again in the pages of these *Oil Notes*. The deeply buried oil reservoirs are as well-concealed as the slaves hidden within a ship's hold. It is as if humanity still hasn't awakened to the fact that the sources of power that maintain it are neither neutral nor free of cost.

Existential causes of repression

The final cause of repression is existential. We would be unable to live, breathe, move, or work, but for the fact that we have captured energy that we can absorb and digest. Our dependence on our environment is total in this respect. Every day, we gather our ration of carbohydrates, proteins and lipids from the living things around us. Should this movement cease, we would starve. Desire is no longer possible when energy is in short supply, and this is why our most basic, fundamental necessity, is that of fuel, first for our bodies, and, secondarily, for our machines. *Energy is the possibility of desire*: this is our basic existential truth. It is not insignificant that the term *libido* refers as much to desire as it does to a form of psychic energy.

The implications of this are numerous. For we who desire do not always like to contemplate what it is that makes our desires possible. Desiring has a price, just as living does. Energy is the result of a predation. The engine of my desire is the *negation* of something else, to use the Hegelian term. Alimentation, which is the way in which human beings procure energy, depends on the slaughter of poultry or sheep, or the harvesting of grain. Living beings inevitably ingest the energy of other living beings, whose lives they negate in the process. Likewise, in earlier times when the energy of slaves was exploited, or even today when we burn fuel, our gain depends on a loss somewhere else. The act of living is not a neutral operation, but a continual siphoning off of external energy which living beings capture and use for their own benefit. This is what we repress: this original, fundamental negation, which could also be called *the cost of living*. It is a biological truth, which, even if no moral interpretation is attached to it, still orients the habitual thought processes of human beings, who prefer not to be constantly reminded that we are the most voracious of all predators, and that the price of our desires is the negation of other wills.

In an age of clear consciences, this truth can be hard to swallow. It must, however, be always at the back of our minds, or else we risk perpetuating a false vision of humanity as an angelic collection of pure spirits, capable of living in energetic harmony. This may be a utopia worth striving toward, but it has nothing to do with our starting position. For humankind is voracious, greedy, dependant and predatory. Maintaining our body temperature at 98.6 degrees Fahrenheit and keeping our brains alert and active requires an enormous intake of energy. Our society masks this as much as it can. Just as the procurement of oil largely escapes our notice and the production of nuclear energy is kept far from the public eye, likewise the immense slaughterhouses, the teaming fish farm pools, and the warehouses full of chickens that will never see the light of day remain at a distance, disguised or hidden. Our backs are turned to all our sources of energy. We could not stand, for example, to see the things that writer Isabelle Sorente describes in her novel *180 jours* (*180 Days*)—the title refers to the duration of a pig's life, from its birth to its final desperate squeal. The rhythm of industrial carnage, the suffering of the livestock workers, the peculiar status of this meat which only becomes "visible" to us once it is wrapped in plastic; none of this escapes the view of Sorente's protagonist, a philosophy professor who has resolved to *see* for himself.[14] But what stamina is required to procure the necessary authorization, what tenacity and what discipline just to keep from looking away. Ordinarily, we avert our gaze, not only out of disgust, but more fundamentally, as a sign of our inability to consciously acknowledge this daily holocaust in which we are complicit and upon which we depend.

Denial is a defence mechanism. We humans cannot bear to be made aware of our own cruelty. But in averting our eyes, we also seek to deny

[14] I. Sorente, *180 jours*, Paris, Lattès, 2013.

our animal nature, for this cruelty is, from the start, the logical corollary of the biological fact that a living thing must consume other living things in order to survive. Under technocapitalism, of course, this biological fact translates into a global factory farming enterprise in which animals are deliberately brought into the world to provide energy for one billion people—six billion others haven't yet been invited to join the party. The enormity of the numbers must not mask the fact that behind these consumer figures are individual human beings, often well intentioned, sometimes even highly sophisticated and politically aware.

Bringing something back to consciousness that has long been repressed requires tact. The error would be to pass judgement too swiftly, or worse, to resort to wholesale condemnation, which would only add moral short-sightedness to an involuntary cultural blindness. Reality must not be more than we can bear. Nietzsche had some apposite comments on this subject, to the effect that exceptional minds are distinguished by the truths that they are able to countenance without looking away. We must recognize that, from the starting point of an already voracious and predatory biological reality, we have progressed to become profligate consumers of energy, and that our energy dependence has become our problem. But we must not, in our agitation, look too hastily for a speedy "solution" . . . The impulse to try to resolve all our problems is understandable, but in this case, it would be ill-advised and ideologically motivated. Philosophy does not exist to resolve problems. It seeks first to understand them, to locate them within a broader context, to untangle their threads. For every question, it tries to discern what does and does not depend on us, how much is a matter of interpretation, how much is based in fact, and how much is a confusing mixture of the two. Understanding is already a form of liberation. Elucidation is a victory in and of itself. Moreover, philosophy is not so naive as to uncritically embrace "solutions" . . . It is more inclined to distrust them, aware that what passes for a solution often involves the complete destruction of whatever was considered problematic. In any case, being human is not a problem. It is a problematic desire, which is quite different.

Dialectic of energy and desire

In the beginning is desire. Living things are driven by impulses, urges, needs, and yearnings. Here, words are used to quickly demarcate boundaries, and each philosophical school has its own way of speaking. But behind the words, their sights are set on the same reality. A tendency to grow and develop is encoded within the dark, miraculous blueprint of life itself, spurring all living beings to exist and go on existing. To live is to have the will to live, as Schopenhauer put it. To be alive is to be shot through with the blind, natural force from which being arises. Some call it "God." Spinoza called it "*Natura naturans*." Jonas spoke of the "Phenomenon of Life." All of these words are like X-rays that seek to penetrate the colourful, fluctuating surface of phenomena, to capture the fundamental process that lies beneath. For our purposes here, we will refer to it as "desire."

This is the point of departure from which we must construct the link between energy and the individual. Desire seeks the means for its own fulfillment, and the first of these means is energy. An embryo is coded for growth: that is its core program, its desire, its will, which it can only realize by absorbing nutrition from the placenta and converting it into energy. Energy makes possible the fulfillment of desire.

In human affairs, too, desire comes first. One person wants to write a book, another wants to go for a walk, or to work. But does each of them have enough energy? That is the first question. For it is our reserves of physical or mental fortitude that allow us to turn our volitions into realities. However much I may wish to teach a class, if I do not have the capacity to get up and speak, the wish will remain unfulfilled. Energy is the means of fulfilling desire.

Things become more interesting as the relationship between human energy and desire grows more complex. An encounter between them is always a noteworthy occasion. Human beings seldom have two days in a row in which their energy levels and degree of health remain constant. Variation is the rule. Energy is always something new, the product of a complex alchemy of nourishment, atmosphere, mood, and relationships.

Above all, it is not a neutral medium. While it may permit the fulfillment of a desire, it never does so in the manner of a formal condition, that simply has to be met. It is a material condition, active and efficacious, always unique, and different each time. This means that human energy transforms desires, even as it fulfills them. It modulates, conditions, and sometimes sparks a metamorphosis. The energy deployed in the service of teaching a class will determine the way the class proceeds, giving the lecturer's words more assurance and conviction, which may sometimes engender the creation of something genuinely novel. If we liken desire to an intention, energy resembles the circumstances of its fulfillment. But well we know that our intentions are very rarely carried out exactly as planned. We can mentally prepare for a meeting, rehearsing what we plan to say, and even conducting the entire conversation in our heads beforehand. But reality always surprises us, and often turns out to be more complex than anything we might have tried to anticipate. One word or one look may be all it takes to derail the conversation, taking it in an entirely different direction from the dialogue we had carefully rehearsed and moving it into uncharted territory. These modifications to the original plan attest to the reality of the interaction, which must take into account the perspectives of both interlocutors, not just the fantasy of a single individual. It is only authoritarian powers, in reality, that can never be thrown off course. They follow the routes they have fixed for themselves, never diverted from their objectives. This is what makes them tiresome, callous and crude. Finesse consists of negotiating with reality, not imposing one's fantasies upon it.

It is by means of this type of negotiation that human energy modifies the desires it serves. We never truly realize our desires. We transform them, depending on the means we find to make them concrete. Otherwise, we would be automatons, programmed to run the same code in the same way, regardless of the circumstances. As it is, we are guided by the forces and the means available to us, to such an extent that we are more inclined to do what we know ourselves to be capable of, rather than what we actually desire. The means govern us. We could construct an entire typology based on this observation. From the lazy types who give priority to their fatigue, to the aimless wanderers who drift along on shifting tides of energy, to the can-do types who somehow always find the resources to realize their goals and the ones who wish to change but no longer have the necessary resolve, we can assemble a richly varied cast of characters. In fact, Balzac has already done it for us in his novels. His *Comédie humaine* is the story of the encounters between the desires of these individuals and the energy each expends in pursuit of them.

From human energy to technical energy, there is continuity at first, then a split, and a surge in power. The principle is still the same: desire comes first, and then energy, as the means of its fulfillment, modulates it and transforms it. The intention to travel across a continent is the initial impetus. Gasoline, burned and converted into kinetic energy by an engine, makes the journey possible. But this energy is still not neutral. It is paid for, captured, coveted. Unlike human energy, it has no upper limit set by the body. External to the individual, it is available in unlimited supply. If there is a split at this point between the two types of energy, it is because technical energy is quantitatively incommensurate with human energy. To be sure, we can state that a cup of oil is equivalent to the amount of physical energy exerted by a human labourer over the course of four months, which gives us a point of comparison. But while the calculation is possible, the difference in scale is radical. Far more powerful than our physical strength, technical energy fulfills desires that did not previously exist. We have only to experience the force of acceleration that glues us to our seats as our jet plane takes off to appreciate this. This energy has effects of its own. Conditioning our desires, it ultimately determines them. It transforms them to such an extent that it winds up recreating them. The postmodern experience is one in which our desires are invented by the energies available to us. Did I really want to make that journey? Or did the energetic possibility of taking it, of purchasing it—since money is another fundamental energy—give rise to the desire? Which comes first, technical energy or human will? Having long repressed the question of means, the

Humanists assumed that human desires remained sovereign. But energy is humanity's collective unconscious, and it must be conceded that it is often the co-author of our actions. Our energy transforms that which we desire. What rational-minded human being would ever have thought it possible to destroy an entire Japanese city with a single bomb, had there been no access to nuclear energy? We believe that we are in control, but in reality, it is often our energy that drives our actions.

The complex dialectic of desire and energy undergoes a reversal comparable to that of the master and slave dialectic. Energy, the means of fulfilling desire, takes on so much importance that it transforms, modifies, and sometimes unseats desire. In Kojève's reading of Hegel's *Phenomenology of Spirit*, the slave ultimately determines the master's consciousness, since the master requires the regard of an inferior in order to exist. Likewise, our relationships with oil, gas or electricity have undergone a reversal. Energy, the slave *par excellence*, has progressed from the literal enslavement of Antiquity, when shackled prisoners of war manned the oars in ships' galleys and ground grain in the mills, toward a future that aligns with Kojève's logic, dictating that the inferior is the one who holds the real power. Our desires, if ever they were in control, must recognize that in today's reality, they are radically dependant on gallons of fuel to which they previously gave no thought.

But the most significant reversal takes place when energy itself becomes the object of our desire. This creates an infinite loop. What had been the means becomes an end. Energy, which had been a tool to serve desire, has grown so powerful, so precious, so capable of effecting transformation, that *it*, rather than that which it makes possible, has become the thing sought after. Desire and energy now merge together. They have become almost indistinguishable. Oil is what our civilization covets. Having been the means of our desire, it has also become its object. We seek energy for energy's sake, the way some people lust after money for money's sake. The reversal results in the identification of means and ends.

Nietzsche predicted this. He who studied the writings of energy physicists while developing his own doctrine[15] and pondered the fact that this notion enables us to leave behind a static materialism in favour of a dynamic, polemical reality. In an unprecedented manner, he ushered in the advent of an unprecedented desire: the desire for energy, otherwise known as the will to power. Before him, the things desired fell into classical categories: to rule, to understand, to create, to live. Power was a condition and a means for accomplishing these activities, but it was not the ultimate objective. Yet, Nietzsche's prognosis is that the alleged purpose of government, which was, according to the classical model, the welfare of the people, would fade away in favour of the power that ruling bestows upon the ruler. His disdain for the weak and the masses, his virile cult of the strong is rooted in this simple question: who has the power? Likewise, the ostensible goal of creation—the work that is created—tends to recede into the background, while the power of the creator and the energy, or "health" of the artist, in Nietzsche's terms, take on primary significance. That which the artist must desire is power, which is yet another name for energy. He must come to desire, so to speak, so that his desire will have the energy necessary for existence. As for the determination of what should be desired—which was the object of Socrates' meditation—we seem to have lost track of it. The important thing is to desire it powerfully! If we agree to replace "will" with "desire" and "power" with "energy," the will to power is, indeed, the desire for energy, which just happens to be the preoccupation of big oil companies, nuclear power plant operators, and all those embroiled in the geopolitics of oil distribution.

Nietzscheism provided the first, vigorous expression of the reversal heralding the thirst for energy, which is now a defining characteristic of our modern world, demonstrating the challenge that Nietzsche posed and still poses to philosophical conventions. He dared to venture out alone. He exposed the hypocrisy of established theories. He was

[15] A. Kremer-Marietti, *Nietzsche et l'énergie de la puissance,* www.dogma.lu.

not afraid to watch the ground open up before him as the idols tumbled down one by one. He was the educator of our disillusionment, the explorer of a new, open terrain, and while he did not map its contours, he was the first to announce its existence. The will to power that he sketched abstractly has become so omnipresent, so often parroted in technological, military, and financial circles, and used as the rallying cry of so many despicable scoundrels over the course of the twentieth century, that even Nietzsche himself might well have been disgusted by this spectacle. At no other point in history have human beings been as drunk on power as they are today. They gorge upon it shamelessly. This isn't the way Nietzsche imagined it. He envisioned a different kind of power; his writings leave no doubt on this point. He had in mind something milder, the quiet vigour of a few strong, stolid individuals, whose power would have been the counterpoint to a particular morality. There is no doubt that the will to power, as construed by our civilization (and as misappropriated by Nazism) is infinitely far removed from Nietzsche's fantasy. But there is also no doubt that this will to power remains the mantra of our power-hungry world. Heidegger understood this. In his lectures on *Nietzsche*, he argued that the will to power, feeding recursively on its own hunger, ran the risk of taking itself as its only goal, thus becoming a "will to will." Is this not an apt description of our current system, which strives to become boundary-less, or in other words, to desire nothing beyond itself?

Post-burnout transition

It is the dominance of this will to power that justifies the classification of burnout as a pathology of civilization. It is not only an individual disorder that afflicts those who have failed to adapt to the system, or become too invested in it, or unable to effectively limit their professional commitments. It is also a mirror disorder that reflects certain unsustainable values within our society: its cult of excess, of performance, of maximization, augmented by technologies that impose their temporal rhythms on human beings.

What is burnout, if not a consequence of these energetic systems running amok? The symptoms of fatigue, anxiety, unmanageable stress, depersonalization and feelings of incompetence paint the portrait of a group of people who have given too much, without getting what they need. They have neglected themselves, often because they had no other choice.

In this context, it becomes urgently necessary that we begin to reflect on transition—from the Latin *trans-ire*, literally, to go beyond. In many domains, whether political, energetic, environmental or technological, the word "transition" refers to efforts to find a new way of envisioning change. For it has become clear that neither techno-capitalism, nor earlier ideals of "revolution" are capable of providing a satisfactory conception of change, given what is now at stake.[16]

Transitions, be they energetic, democratic, or demographic, open up space in which to forge a new relationship with the future. Within this space, different preferences can be asserted; subtle progress—more profound than the useful progress to which we are accustomed—can at last receive its due. Within this space, our planet may no longer be perceived as a collection of resources to be exploited, but as a place where human beings come face to face with the mystery of existence and are forced to grapple with fundamental questions: what influence do we have over human evolution? What must we change to keep everything from changing for the worse?

Michel Serres invented the character of Petite Poucette to represent today's hyper-connected younger generation. Sitting on her Ikea sofa, eyes glued to the new i-Phone she ordered from Amazon, she symbolizes the immediate impact of progress on the individual. But some Cartesian evil genius might yet come to introduce an element of doubt into

16 The "pact with technology" that we alluded to earlier constitutes a part of this transition. For a more thorough development of this notion, especially with regard to energetic transition and the construction of a new mentality, see P. Chabot, *L'âge des transitions*, Paris, PUF, 2015.

her comfortable existence, informing her of the deplorable working conditions, environmental destruction, and damaged health that are the hidden price of her comfort. The end of innocence casts us into a state of divided consciousness: we want to continue to enjoy the useful inventions that bring us pleasure, but their hidden cost is unacceptable. We must therefore make a choice between guilt and imagination: how can we mitigate the damage caused by progress, without taking a step backwards? Opening our eyes to the consequences of our way of life is the first step toward transition.

The intellectual challenge of transition is imagining a future beyond global burnout, by striving to establish a more sustainable way of life. The evolution of our mentalities now becomes a crucial issue. And the pursuit of balance between the useful progress that dominates our present world and subtle progress, too often neglected, is equally crucial, if we want this era to reveal itself not as the prelude to a catastrophe, but as an opportunity for reinvention that gives rise to a new humanism, rooted in a world that acknowledges and celebrates the mystery of existence.

Author's Acknowledgments

This book is the product of many discussions, notably with a number of people who themselves suffered through the ordeal of burnout. I offer them my sincere gratitude. Thank you also to my colleagues at the Institut des Hautes Études en Communications Sociales (IHECS) in Brussels, who contribute to creating a very congenial work environment, and who have expanded my understanding of numerous topics.

My editors, Laurent de Sutter and Paul Garapon, are always keenly discerning, and Claire Lagarde's invaluable assistance was of instrumental importance.

For this English edition, I also wish to thank Patricia Pisters and Bernd Herzogenrath, who have paid me the great honour of welcoming this text into their collection. The advice they offered has been invaluable. Many thanks as well to the Bloomsbury editorial team. As far as the translation is concerned, working with Aliza Krefetz is always a true pleasure, as well as an assurance of genuine *quality*.

This book was the basis for a documentary film, "Burning out," directed by Jérôme le Maire. I extend my warmest thanks to him, and to the producer, Arnauld de Battice of AT Productions. The experience of moving from conceptual thought to cinematic narration was unforgettable. The depth of their questions and the discussions they generated were equaled only by the quality of the encounters we had at the Hôpital Saint-Louis, in Paris, where the entire film was shot, in showing and explaining, from the perspective of health professionals, the realities of working in a large hospital today.

Some of the questions explored in this book were first raised at the *Mardis de la Philosophie* lecture series, thanks to Amélie d'Oultremont and Martine Legein. Many thanks also to François Lagarde, Franck Pierobon, Éric de Bellefroid, Judith Delville, Gillian Lefevre, Geoffroy De Ligne, Elisabeth Leijnse, Michèle Noiret and my brother Pierre-Axel, as well as my parents and my entire family. My children gave me the opportunity to disprove the old adage *Aut libri aut liberi* (either books or children), which is surely cause for celebration. My wife Vinci gave me the keys for addressing many questions.

Translator's Acknowledgments

Many thanks to Pascal Chabot for his encouragement throughout the translation process. Thank you also to Sharon Krefetz, Elliott Krefetz, and Suckbir Pal Singh Sangha for their support, and to James Maraniss, for turning me on to translation.

Bibliography

Apuleius, *The Golden Ass, or Metamorphoses*, trans. E.J. Kenney, London, Penguin Books, 2004.

Bachelard G., *Psychoanalysis of Fire*, trans. Alan C.M. Ross, Boston, Beacon Press, 1964.

Bass R., *Oil Notes*, Lincoln, University of Nebraska Press, 2012.

Baudelaire C, *Les fleurs du mal*, Paris, Gallimard, 1972.

Baudelaire C, *Fusées*, Paris, Gallimard, 1986.

Baudelaire C, *Mon coeur mis à nu*, Paris, Gallimard, 1986.

Baudelaire C, *Le spleen de Paris*, Paris, Flammarion, 1987.

Bergson, H. *L'énergie spirituelle*, Paris, PUF, 1959 (1st edition 1919).

Burger A., "Comment devenir un meilleur professionnel en se protégeant [How to become a better professional by protecting yourself]," in *Repère Social*, No. 19, July 2000.

Caillé A. (ed.), *La quête de reconnaissance. Nouveau phénomène social total* [*The Quest for Recognition: a Completely New Social Phenomenon*], Paris, La Découverte, 2007.

Cassian, *The Twelve Books of John Cassian on the Institutes of the Coenobia, and the Remedies for the Eight Principal Faults*. Translated by Edgar C.S. Gibson, from *A Select Library of Nicene and Post-Nicene Fathers of the Christian Church, Second Series*, Vol. 11. New York, 1894.

Chabot P., *Les sept stades de la philosophie* [*The Seven Stages of Philosophy*], Paris, PUF, 2011.

Chabot P., *The Philosophy of Simondon*, London, Bloomsbury, 2013, translated by Graeme Kirkpatrick and Aliza Krefetz.

Chabot P., *L'âge des transitions*, Paris, PUF, 2015.

Chabot P., *Exister, résister. Ce qui dépend de nous*, Paris, PUF, 2017.

Chevalier J. and Gheerbrant A., *Dictionnaire des symbols* [*Dictionary of Symbols*], Paris, Robert Laffont, 1982.

Crawford M.B., *Shop Class as Soulcraft: An Inquiry into the Value of Work*, New York, Penguin Press, 2009.

Debeir J.C., Deléage J.P. and Hémery D., in *Une histoire de l'énergie*, Paris, Flammarion, 2013.

Dejours C., *Travail vivant. 2. Travail et emancipation* [*Work and Emancipation*], Paris, Payot, 2009.

Dejours C. (ed.), *Observations cliniques en psychopathologie du travail* [*Clinical and Psychopathological Observations of Work*], Paris, PUF, 2010.

Delbrouck M., *Comment traiter le burn-out* [*How to Treat Burnout*], Brussels, De Boeck, 2011.

Deleuze G. and Guattari F., *Anti-Oedipus*, trans. Robert Hurley, Mark Seem, and Helen R. Lane, Viking, London, 1984.

Delfour J.-J., *La condition nucléaire. Réflexions sur la situation atomique de l'humanité*, Montreuil, Editions L'échappée, 2014.

de Kerangal M., *Birth of a Bridge*, trans. Jessica Moore, Vancouver, Talonbooks, 2014.

Desbordes J.-P., *Management circus. Une critique du management à l'époque postmoderne* [*Management Circus: a Critique of Management in the Postmodern Age*], Arles, Actes Sud, 2012.

des Isnards A. and Zuber T., *L'open space m'a tuer* [*Open Space Killed Me*], Paris, Le Livre de Poche, 2008.

Dictionnaire de théologie catholique [*Dictionary of Catholic Theology*], Article on "Paresse [Sloth]," by E. Vansteenberghe, Letouzey Ed., 1932, Vol. XI, Part 2.

Echenoz J., *Lightning* [*Des éclairs*], trans. Linda Coverdale, New York, The New Press, 2011.

Everard A., *Guide du burn-out*, Paris, Albin Michel, 2017.

Fain M., Cournut J., Enriquez E. and Cifali M., *Les trois métiers impossibles* [*The Three Impossible Professions*], Paris, Les Belles Lettres, 1987.

Forthomme B., *De l'acédie monastique à l'anxio-dépression. Histoire philosophique de la transformation d'un vice en pathologie* [*From Monastic Acedia to Anxiety and Depression: a Philosophical History of the Transformation of a Vice into a Pathology*], Paris, Les empêcheurs de penser en rond, 2000.

Freud S., "Analysis Terminable and Interminable," in *International Journal of Psycho-Analysis*, Vol. 18, Psychoanalytic Electronic Publishing, 2012.

Freudenberger H. and North G., *Women's Burnout*, London, Penguin, 1985.

Freudenberger H.J. and Richardson G., *Burn-Out. The High Cost of High Achievement*, London, Arrow Edition, 1985 (1st edition New York, Doubleday).

Ghesquier-Pourcin D., *Ostwald et le monisme*, in D. Ghesquier-Pourcin, M. Guedj, G. Gohau and M. Party, *Energie, science et philosophie. Les formes de l'énergétisme et leur influence sur la pensée*, Paris, Hermann, 2010.

Greene G., *A Burnt-Out Case*, New York, Viking Press, 1961.

Greene G., *In Search of a Character: Two African Journals.* New York, Viking Press, 1961.

Guénon R., *Le règne de la quantité et les signes des temps* [*The Reign of Quantity and the Signs of the Times*], Paris, Gallimard, "NRF tradition," 1945.

Guéricault V., *La fatigue émotionnelle et physique des mères* [*The Physical and Emotional Fatigue of Mothers*], Paris, Odile Jacob, 2004.

Han B.-C., *The Burnout Society*, Stanford, Stanford University Press, 2015.

Honneth A., *The I in We: Studies in the Theory of Recognition*, Cambridge, Polity Press, 2012.

Hottois G. and Missa J.N., *L'humain et ses préfixes*, Paris, Vrin, 2016.

Huxley A., "Accidie," in *On the Margin*, London, Chatto & Windus, 1923.

Jung, C.G. "On Psychic Energy" in *On the Nature of the Psyche*, Princeton, Princeton University Press, 1960.

Jünger E., *Zahlen und Götter* [*Numbers and Gods*], Stuttgart, Klett-Cotta, 1975.

Kraft U., "Burned Out," *Scientific American Mind*, June–July 2006.

Lakoff G. and Johnson M., *Metaphors We Live By*, Chicago, University of Chicago Press, 1980.

Martel P., *Burn-out*, Biarritz, Atlantica, 2010.

Maslach C. and Leiter M., *The Truth about Burnout.* San Francisco, Wiley, 1997.

Mayoux J.-J., Introduction to the French edition of J. Conrad, *Heart of Darkness* [*Au coeur des ténèbres*], Paris, Flammarion, 1989.

Meesters P. and Peters S., *Vaincre l'épuisement professionnel* [*Overcoming Professional Exhaustion*], Paris, Robert Laffont, 2007.

Molinier P., *L'énigme de la femme active. Sexe, égoïsme et compassion* [*The Enigma of the Working Woman: Sex, Egoism, and Compassion*], Paris, Payot, 2003.

Molinier P., *Les enjeux psychiques du travail* [*The Psychological Stakes of Work*], Paris, Payot, 2006.

Nietzsche F., *Beyond Good and Evil*, London, Penguin Books, 1973.

Nuttin J., "Adaptation," in *Encyclopédie Universalis*, Paris, 1990, tome 1.

O'Neill J., *Prodigal Genius: The Life of Nikola Tesla*, New York, Cosimo, Inc., 2006.

Péguy C., *L'Argent* [*On Money*], Paris, Éditions des Équateurs, 2008.

Pélegrin-Genel E., *Des souris dans un labyrinthe. Décrypter les ruses et manipulations de nos espaces quotidiens* [*Rats in a Maze: Decrypting the Ruses and Manipulations of our Everyday Spaces*], Paris, La Découverte, 2010.

Pezé M., *Ils ne mouraient pas tous mais tous étaient frappés* [*They Didn't All Die, but All were Stricken*], Paris, Flammarion, 2010.

Quintreau L., *Marge brute*, Paris, Denoël, 2006.

Richter F., *Under Ice* (trans. David Tushingham), S. Fischer Verlag, 2004.

Rosa H., *Social Acceleration: A New Theory of Modernity*, trans. Jonathan Trejo-Mathys, New York, Columbia University Press, 2013.

Scherrer J., *La Fatigue*. Paris, PUF, 1989.

Simondon G., *L'individu et sa genèse physico-biologique* [*The Physico-Biological Genesis of the Individual*], Grenoble, Million, 1988.

Simondon G., *Du mode d'existence des objets techniques* [*On the Mode of Existence of Technical Objects*], Paris, Aubier, 1958 (ed. 1989).

Sloterdijk P., *Falls Europa erwacht* [*If Europe Awakes*], Frankfurt, Suhrkamp, 1994.

Sloterdijk P., *You Must Change Your Life*, trans. Wieland Hoban, Polity Press, Cambridge, 2013.

Solomon A., *The Noonday Demon: An Atlas of Depression*, New York, Simon and Schuster, 2001.

Sorente I., *Addiction générale* [*General Addiction*], Paris, Jean-Claude Lattès, 2011.

Sorente I., *180 jours*, Paris, Lattès, 2013.

Styron W., *Darkness Visible: A Memoir of Madness*. New York, Random House, 1990.

Tavares G.M., *Apprendre à prier à l'ère de la technique*. Paris, Viviane Hamy, 2010.

Teilhard de Chardin, P. *L'énergie humaine*, Paris, Seuil, 1962.

Terence M., *Le devenir du nombre*, Paris, Stock, 2012.

Valéry P., *Dance and the Soul*, trans. Dorothy Bussy, London, J. Lehmann, 1951.

Woolf V., *The Waves*, Oxford, Oxford University Press, 1992.

Woolf V., *A Room of One's Own*, New York: Harcourt, 2005.

Worms F., *Revivre*, Paris, Flammarion, 2012.

Index